Farah Azouzi
Houyem Said Laatiri
Olfa Bouallègue

Antibiotic resistance

Farah Azouzi
Houyem Said Laatiri
Olfa Bouallègue

Antibiotic resistance

Evolution of antibiotic resistance in high-risk nosocomial infection departments in Tunis

ScienciaScripts

Imprint
Any brand names and product names mentioned in this book are subject to trademark, brand or patent protection and are trademarks or registered trademarks of their respective holders. The use of brand names, product names, common names, trade names, product descriptions etc. even without a particular marking in this work is in no way to be construed to mean that such names may be regarded as unrestricted in respect of trademark and brand protection legislation and could thus be used by anyone.

Cover image: www.ingimage.com

This book is a translation from the original published under ISBN 978-620-3-42364-8.

Publisher:
Sciencia Scripts
is a trademark of
Dodo Books Indian Ocean Ltd., member of the OmniScriptum S.R.L Publishing group
str. A.Russo 15, of. 61, Chisinau-2068, Republic of Moldova Europe
Printed at: see last page
ISBN: 978-620-4-05242-7

Evolution of antibiotic resistance in high-risk hospital wards in Tunisia

Farah Azouzi, Nihel Haddad, Asma Ben Cheikh, Walid Naija, Houyem Said Laatiri, Olfa Bouallègue.

Summary

Abbreviations

BGN: Gram-negative bacilli

HRB: highly resistant bacteria

ESBL: extended-spectrum betalactamases

MDR: multi-drug resistant bacteria

CA-SFM: Antibiogram Committee of the French Society of Microbiology

CDC: Center for Disease Control and Prevention

CLIN: Comité de Lutte Contre les Infections Nosocomiales

E-BLSE: extended-spectrum betalactamase-producing enterobacteria

ECBU: cytobacteriological examination of urine

ECDC: European Center for Disease Control and Prevention

EUCAST: The European Committee on Antimicrobial Susceptibility Testing

HCAI: Healthcare Associated Infections

LART: Antibio-resistance in Tunisia

ONERBA: National Observatory of the Epidemiology of Bacterial Resistance to Antibiotics

PACS: Services Competitiveness Support Project

VAP: mechanically ventilated lung disease

PDP: Protected Distal Picking

POG: postoperative department of the general surgery

MRSA: methicillin-resistant *Staphylococcus aureus*

XDR: Extensively Drug Resistant

Introduction

Introduction

The use of substances with antimicrobial activity dates back thousands of years even before the era of modern antibiotic therapy. As early as 2500 BC, the ancient Egyptians used myrrh as a topical wound treatment. Hippocrates also reported the therapeutic properties of myrrh in 400 BC. The Romans later used it in addition to barbarum to treat septic conditions (1).

The modern era of antibiotics owes much to the work of Rudolf Emmerich and Oscar Low who discovered in the 19th century that the "pyocyanase" or green bacteria that covered patients' bandages inhibited the growth of other microbes. The modern era of antimicrobials really began with Paul Ehrlich who, at the same time, noticed that some of the stains used for tissue observation were toxic to certain bacteria.

Alexander Fleming published in 1929 the antimicrobial effect of *Penicillium* on several bacterial species and thus discovered penicillin (2). But long before him, several observations in the 19th century already reported the ability of molds to inhibit bacterial growth. These were even used by Arab horsemen to treat siege irritations and Ernest Duchesne confirmed that they were *Penicillium notatum* cultures and used them to successfully treat typhoid induced in guinea pigs (3).

The golden age of antibiotics began in the early 1940s with the use of penicillin in the clinic and the discovery of streptomycin and its use to treat Gram-negative bacilli. The first penicillinase-producing strains of staphylococci soon appeared and within ten years most hospital strains became resistant to penicillin.

In forty years, more than 20 classes of antibiotics have been developed and each time a new antibiotic was marketed, new resistance mechanisms spread (1).

Nowadays, bacterial resistance to antibiotics is a real public health problem. The worldwide spread of multidrug-resistant bacteria is no longer limited to hospitals but also to the community, where it is no longer unusual to diagnose infections with extended-spectrum Betalactamase (ESBL)-producing Enterobacteriaceae (4).

This pandemic has put all national and international bodies on alert. The World Health Organization (WHO) has made this problem a priority and in February 2017 published a list of resistant bacteria for which there is an urgent need to develop new antibiotics. Bacteria categorized as critical are carbapenem-resistant *Acinetobacter baumannii*, carbapenem-resistant *Pseudomonas aeruginosa*, and carbapenem- and/or 3rd generation cephalosporin-resistant Enterobacteriaceae (5). The Centers for Disease Control and Prevention (CDC) and WHO recently organized Antibiotic Awareness Week (6). Indeed, bacterial resistance to antibiotics is a problem that concerns not only health actors but also the general public. Collective collaboration is essential to preserve antibiotics and avoid returning to the pre-antibiotic era.

Our country is not spared from this problem either and different studies report high rates of bacterial resistance to different classes of antibiotics (7-9). The Tunisian network L'Antibio-Résistance en Tunisie (LART) gathers several microbiology laboratories and has the mission to monitor the evolution of resistance to antibiotics in the main bacterial species (10).

The microbiology laboratory plays an essential role in the detection of bacterial resistance and in the indication of appropriate antibiotic therapy, but also in the prevention of the horizontal spread of multi-resistant germs in collaboration with the clinical services and the hygiene service.

Our hospital, which has a surgical vocation, is particularly concerned by the growing problem of multi-resistant bacteria, given the frequency of nosocomial infections. It is within the framework of the monitoring of bacterial antibiotic resistance that we have carried out this work, the main objectives of which are

- describe the bacterial ecology of four at-risk departments at Sahloul Hospital

- determine the level of resistance of the main species isolated

Materials and methods

Materials and methods

- Operational definition of variables :

o Definition of the term evolution :

We define resistance trends as any trend of increasing or decreasing rates of bacterial resistance to the antibiotics tested during a given time period or when comparing data from two or more different years (11).

o Definition of bacterial resistance to antibiotics :

In our work, we were interested in the acquired resistance of bacteria to antibiotics.

A bacterium is said to be resistant to an antibiotic if the inhibition diameter around this antibiotic is less than the threshold diameter or if the MIC of this antibiotic is higher than the threshold value quoted in the CA-SFM/EUCAST (12).

Strains with intermediate resistance were considered as resistant in this study. The level of resistance to the tested antibiotics was therefore divided into two: susceptible and resistant strains (intermediate and resistant).

o Definition of multidrug resistance :

A bacterium is said to be multidrug resistant (MDR) if it is resistant to at least three families of antibiotics (13).

o Definition of an XDR (Extensively Drug Resistant) bacterium:

An XDR bacterium remains sensitive to only two or fewer molecules (13).

o Definition of a pan or total resistant strain:

It is a bacterium that is not sensitive to any antibiotic molecule (13).

o BMR monitored at Sahloul Hospital (5):

Nine BMR are actively monitored at Sahloul Hospital: cefotaxime-resistant *K. pneumoniae*, ertapenem-resistant *K. pneumoniae*, cefotaxime-resistant *E. coli*, ertapenem-resistant *E. coli*, imipenem-resistant *A. baumannii* resistant to imipenem, ceftazidime-resistant *P. aeruginosa*, imipenem-resistant *P. aeruginosa*, glycopeptide-resistant enterococci and MRSA.

• Location of the study

The Sahloul Hospital of Sousse is composed of 33 medical services including 3 laboratories, a technical platform including radiology services and pharmacy, 10 surgical services, 25 operating rooms and a catheterization room. It has a hospital capacity of 583 authorized beds, but in practice has 684 beds. An average of 2,026 admissions are recorded per year. The surgical resuscitation, medical resuscitation, POG and urology departments have a capacity of 12, 5, 19 and 60 beds respectively.

- ## Type of study :

This is a retrospective descriptive study conducted at the Sahloul University Hospital of Sousse on all non-redundant bacterial strains isolated from samples sent to the microbiology laboratory by the four departments concerned: urology department, surgical resuscitation department, general surgery postoperative department (POG) and medical resuscitation department, and this over a period of seven years extending from January [1,] 2010 to December 31, 2016.

The choice of these four wards was based on the results of a previous thesis carried out in the same laboratory (14) which identified them as being at high risk of BMR infection.

- ## Study population :

Target population: all bacterial strains isolated from samples sent to the microbiology laboratory and coming from all departments of the Sahloul University Hospital.

Source population: This study focused on **all** non-redundant bacterial strains (**exhaustive study**) isolated from samples sent to the microbiology laboratory by four departments of the Sahloul University Hospital: urology department, surgical resuscitation department, general surgery postoperative department (POG) and medical resuscitation department **Statistical unit**: a bacterial strain

Inclusion criteria:

Bacterial strains isolated from samples sent to the microbiology laboratory by the four departments concerned: urology department, surgical resuscitation department, general surgery post-op department (POG) and medical resuscitation department.

Non-inclusion criteria:

Samples from consultations in the above-mentioned departments and duplicates were excluded from the study.

Conduct of the study :

In order to identify the germs and to study their antibiotic resistance at Sahloul Hospital in Sousse, the data collection was based on :

- o **Bacteriological study :**

Bacteria were identified using conventional methods and refined by the use of the Vitek2 automated system.

The evaluation of their antibiotic susceptibility was performed according to the recommendations of the Comité de l'Antibiogramme de la Société Française de Microbiologie

(CA-SMF) from 2010 to 2013 and then according to the recommendations of the CA-SFM/EUCAST (European Committee on Antimicrobial Susceptibility Testing) from 2014 onwards (15-21).

In some cases, additional tests were required:

- Determination of minimum inhibitory concentrations (MIC) by E-test strips

- synergy test: testing for synergy between a beta-lactamase inhibitor-containing antibiotic disc and a third- or fourth-generation cephalosporin or an aztreonam disc for extended-spectrum beta-lactamase (ESBL) production in enterobacteria

- agglutination technique for the detection of PLP2a in methicillin-resistant staphylococci (MRSA)

- use of combined carbapenem+EDTA, carbapenem+boronic acid and carbapenem+clavulanic acid discs to aid in the identification of carbapenemases

o **Data collection :**

1. Data collection procedure

We collected all the antibiograms of the strains isolated from the positive bacteriological samples from the above-mentioned departments retrospectively from the database of our microbiology laboratory (SIR-Scan software and archives).

2. Investigative tools

The data collected for each isolated strain were

- the requesting department: urology, surgical resuscitation, medical resuscitation and POG

- the nature of the sample: ECBU (urine cytobacteriological examination), blood cultures, PDP (protected distal sampling), deep pus, peripheral pus...

- the year of isolation: 2010 to 2016

- the level of resistance to the antibiotics tested: susceptible and resistant (intermediate or resistant).

Duplicates were eliminated manually.

- ## Statistical analysis of data:

The analysis and interpretation of the data was done using SPSS version 22 software. The database identified from SIR-Scan software for the years 2013, 2014 and 2016 was directly opened in SPSS software.

The data for the years 2010 to 2012 and 2015 were manually transcribed into a data collection form and then transferred to SPSS.

1. **Descriptive study**

Categorical variables were summarized by absolute and relative frequencies.

We performed global resistance statistics within the main species of medical interest.

For a given bacterial species, the percentage of resistance to an antibiotic was calculated by dividing the number of non-susceptible bacteria by the number of bacteria tested for that antibiotic.

2. **Analytical study**

The Chi-square test was performed:

- For the comparison of trends in the annual percentages of resistance for the most representative antibiotic/bacterial species pairs. The p could not be calculated if no resistance was noted for a given antibiotic or if at least one cell had a theoretical number of cells <5, the test becoming uninterpretable.

- To investigate whether there is a significant increase in resistance to aminoglycosides and fluoroquinolones in cefotaxime-resistant strains *of E. coh* and *K. pneumoniae compared to* cefotaxime-sensitive strains.

The difference is significant at p<0.05.

- Ethical considerations

In addition to anonymity, there were no special ethical considerations for this study.

Results

Results:

Global epidemiology :

Isolated germs :

A total of 6108 strains were recovered over a seven-year period.

The bacteria isolated were *Escherichia coli* (n=1329, 21.8%), *Klebsiellapneumoniae* (n=992, 16.2%), *Acinetobacter baumannii* (n=763, 12.5%), *Pseudomonas aeruginosa* (n=625, 10.2%), *Enterococcus faecalis* (n=476, 7.8%), *Staphylococcus aureus* (n=366, 6%), *Enterobacter cloacae* (n=313, 5.1%), *Proteus mirabilis* (n=207, 3.4%), and group B streptococci (n=90, 1.5%) (**Figure 1**).

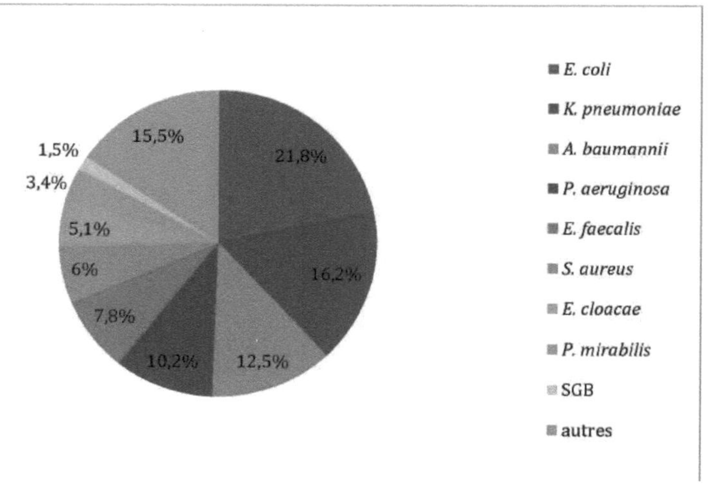

Figure 1: Bacteria isolated

Evolution of the number of isolates by year :

From 2010 to 2016, 488, 1261, 1395, 690, 936, 794 and 544 strains were isolated respectively **(Figure 2)**.

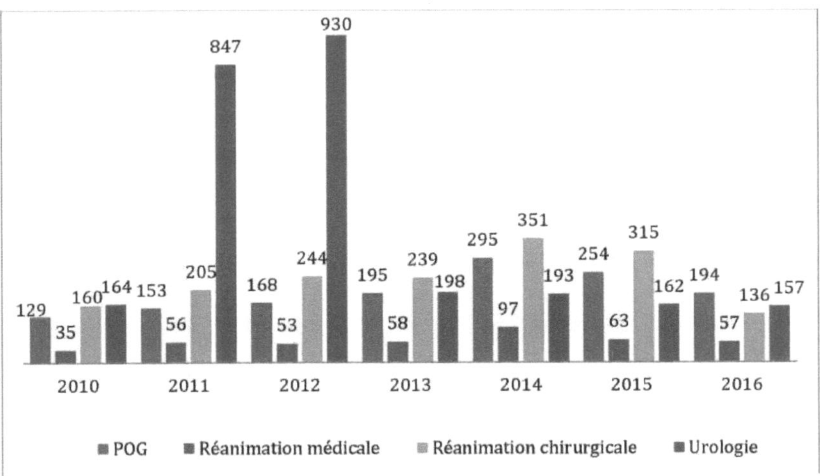

Figure 2: Annual change in the number of isolates

Clinical services involved:

Germs were isolated from urology (n=2651, 43.4%), surgical resuscitation (n=1650, 27%), POG (n=1388, 22.7%) and medical resuscitation (n=419, 6.9%) departments **(Figure 3)**.

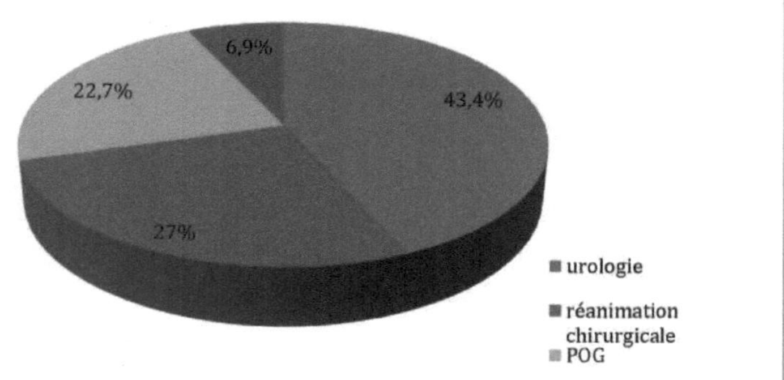

Figure 3: Distribution of isolates by department

Types of samples :

Our strains were isolated from urocultures (n=279, 45.8%), blood cultures (n=1367, 22.4%), medical devices such as catheters, drains and catheters (n=546, 8.9%), protected distal swabs (n=545, 8.9%), deep suppurations (n=442, 7.2%), superficial suppurations (n=98, 1.6%) and ENT swabs (n=91, 1.5%) **(Figure 4)**.

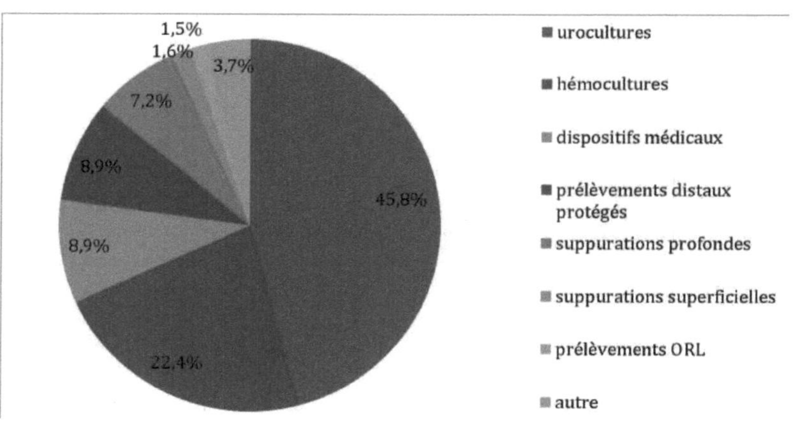

Figure 4: Types of sampling

Annual evolution of antibiotic resistance in the main bacterial species :

The annual evolution of antibiotic resistance for the most frequently isolated bacteria, namely *E. coli, K. pneumoniae, A. baumannii, P. aeruginosa, E. faecalis* and *S. aureus,* is shown in Tables I to VI.

Table I: Annual trends in antibiotic resistance in *E. coli*

	2010 (N=94)	2011 (N=383)	2012 (N=426)	2013 (N=119)	2014 (N=122)	2015 (N=91)	2016 (N=94)	P
Amoxicillin (n/N')	69/94 (73,4%)	253/383 (66,1%)	280/423 (66,2%)	98/119 (82,4%)	99/122 (81,1%)	61/78 (78,2%)	85/93 (91,4%)	<0,001
Amoxicillin-clavulanate (n/N')	39/93 (41,9%)	151/383 (39,4%)	191/426 (44,8%)	66/119 (55,5%)	65/122 (53,3%)	44/78 (56,4%)	37/93 (39,8%)	0,023
Cefoxitin (n/N')	6/94 (6,4%)	19/381 (5%)	1/18 (5,6%)	8/119 (6,7%)	8/122 (6,6%)	4/78 (5,1%)	3/93 (3,2%)	-
Cefotaxime (n/N')	12/94 (12,8%)	61/380 (16,1%)	66/421 (15,7%)	34/118 (28,8%)	49/121 (40,5%)	27/78 (34,6%)	36/93 (38,7%)	<0,001
Imipenem (n/N')	0/93	0/381	0/423	0/119	0/122	0/78	0/91	-
Ertapenem (n/N')	0/5	0/375	0/420	1/119 (0,8%)	0/114	0/78	1/93 (1,1%)	-
Gentamicin (n/N')	16/93 (17,2%)	68/380 (17,9%)	66/425 (15,5%)	29/119 (24,4%)	32/113 (28,3%)	28/78 (35,9%)	27/93 (29%)	<0,001
Amikacin (n/N')	5/94 (5,3%)	20/381 (5,2%)	30/423 (7,1%)	10/119 (8,4%)	18/121 (14,9%)	7/77 (9,1%)	4/93 (4,3%)	0,103
Nalidixic acid (n/N')	23/73 (31,5%)	166/345 (48,1%)	176/387 (45,5%)	-	-	30/46 (65,2%)	60/92 (65,2%)	-
Ofloxacin (n/N')	32/93 (34,4%)	173/383 (45,2%)	194/424 (45,8%)	-	-	49/78 (62,8%)	57/93 (61,3%)	<0,001
Ciprofloxacin (n/N')	28/94 (29,8%)	167/382 (43,7%)	188/424 (44,3%)	52/119 (43,7%)	71/113 (62,8%)	45/78 (57,7%)	57/93 (61,3%)	<0,001
Cotrimoxazole (n/N')	46/93 (49,5%)	195/379 (51,5%)	215/420 (51,2%)	-	-	41/67 (61,2%)	56/93 (60,2%)	0,036
Fosfomycin (n/N')	1/93 (1,1%)	1/380 (0,3%)	2/423 (0,5%)	-	-	0/54	0/92	-
Chloramphenicol (n/N')	10/22 (45,5%)	15/38 (39,5%)	15/47 (31,9%)	1/118 (0,8%)	1/101 (1%)	6/34 (17,6%)	16/92 (17,4%)	-
Colistin (n/N')	0/90	0/376	0/421	0/114	0/121	0/51	-	-

n = number of resistant strains per year

N'= number of strains tested (this number varies by year and by antibiotic tested) N= number of strains isolated per year

Concerning the 285 strains resistant to cefotaxime, 91.9% were also resistant to ciprofloxacin, 65% were resistant to gentamicin. For the strains sensitive to cefotaxime, 97.3% were also sensitive to amikacin. The Pearson Chi-square test was performed with a p less than 0.05 each time.

Table II: Annual trends in antibiotic resistance in *K. pneumoniae*

	2010 (N=78)	2011 (N=214)	2012 (N=222)	2013 (N=150)	2014 (N=133)	2015 (N=124)	2016 (N=71)	P
Amoxicillin-clavulanate (n/N')	78/78 (100%)	213/213 (100%)	116/222 (52,3%)	91/150 (60,7%)	87/133 (65,4%)	76/103 (73,8%)	34/70 (48,6%)	<0,001
Cefoxitin (n/N')	5/77 (6,5%)	17/212 (8%)	0/1	45/150 (30%)	37/132 (28%)	35/103 (34%)	15/70 (21,4%)	-
Cefotaxime (n/N')	37/78 (47,4%)	111/212 (52,4%)	99/220 (45%)	85/150 (56,7%)	70/132 (53%)	63/103 (61,2%)	37/70 (52,9%)	0,079
Imipenem (n/N')	0/78	4/210 (1,9%)	14/221 (6,3%)	33/150 (22%)	29/133 (21,8%)	15/103 (14,6%)	8/69 (11,6%)	<0,001
Ertapenem (n/N')	0/5	4/209 (1,9%)	21/221 (9,5%)	41/148 (27,7%)	36/132 (27,3%)	38/103 (36,9%)	18/69 (26,1%)	-
Gentamicin (n/N')	38/78 (48,7%)	81/210 (38,6%)	88/222 (39,6%)	78/150 (52%)	59/123 (48%)	64/103 (62,1%)	28/70 (40%)	0,022
Amikacin (n/N')	15/78 (19,2%)	30/213 (14,1%)	48/222 (21,6%)	30/150 (20%)	18/131 (13,7%)	28/102 (27,5%)	9/70 (12,9%)	0,624
Nalidixic acid (n/N')	27/42 (64,3%)	93/148 (62,8%)	92/160 (57,5%)	8/27 (29,6%)	13/20 (65%)	51/63 (81%)	38/69 (55,1%)	0,661
Ofloxacin (n/N')	44/78 (56,4%)	127/213 (59,6%)	130/221 (58,8%)	-	-	69/103 (67%)	36/70 (51,4%)	0,820
Ciprofloxacin (n/N')	43/78 (55,1%)	126/213 (59,2%)	128/222 (57,7%)	95/150 (63,3%)	78/126 (61,9%)	66/103 (64,1%)	35/70 (50%)	0,765
Cotrimoxazole (n/N')	34/77 (44,2%)	86/211 (40,8%)	101/221 (45,7%)	-	-	54/89 (60,7%)	29/70 (41,4%)	0,091
Fosfomycin (n/N')	4/75 (5,3%)	18/211 (8,5%)	7/220 (3,2%)	-	-	7/78 (9%)	3/70 (4,3%)	-
Chloramphenicol (n/N')	11/33 (33,3%)	20/66 (30,3%)	24/60 (40%)	8/149 (5,4%)	5/114 (4,4%)	33/75 (44%)	16 /70 (22,9%)	0,332
Colistin (n/N')	0/77	0/208	0/221	0/139	0/128	6/82 (11,8%)	0/12	-

n = number of resistant strains per year

N'= number of strains tested (this number varies by year and by antibiotic tested) N= number of strains isolated per year

Cefotaxime resistant *K. pneumoniae* strains were also resistant to gentamicin, amikacin and ciprofloxacin in 81.3%, 33.8% and 95% of cases respectively. The Pearson Chi-square test was performed with a p of less than 0.05 in each case.

Table III: Annual trends in antibiotic resistance in *A. baumannii*

	2010 (N=55)	2011 (N=51)	2012 (N=143)	2013 (N=114)	2014 (N=163)	2015 (N=139)	2016 (N=98)	P
Ticarcillin (n/N')	54/55 (98,2%)	44/51 (86,3%)	130/140 (92,9%)	111/114 (97,4%)	159/162 (98,1%)	90/92 (97,8%)	96/97 (99%)	-
Ticarcillin-Clavulanate (n/N')	53/54 (98,1%)	42/47 (89,4%)	120/128 (93,8%)	109/112 (97,3%)	135/138 (97,8%)	89/91 (97,8%)	96/97 (99%)	-
Piperacillin (n/N')	54/55 (98,2%)	43/50 (86%)	133/140 (95%)	108/111 (97,3%)	158/162 (97,5%)	71/71 (100%)	2/2 (100%)	-
Piperacillin-Tazobactam (n/N')	54/55 (98,2%)	43/51 (84,3%)	111/122 (91%)	108/113 (95,6%)	149/152 (98%)	70/71 (98,6%)	2/2 (100%)	-
Ceftazidime (n/N')	43/53 (81,1%)	38/48 (79,2%)	127/140 (90,7%)	106/110 (96,4%)	140/159 (88,1%)	86/91 (94,5%)	4/4 (100%)	-
Imipeneme (n/N')	52/55 (94,5%)	38/51 (74,5%)	120/142 (84,5%)	109/114 (95,6%)	158/163 (96,9%)	89/92 (96,7%)	96/97 (99%)	-
Amikacin (n/N')	52/55 (94,5%)	43/50 (86%)	117/142 (82,4%)	108/114 (94,7%)	148/162 (91,4%)	70/92 (76,1%)	82/95 (86,3%)	0,182
Ciprofloxacin (n/N')	46/53 (86,8%)	42/51 (82,4%)	137/143 (95,8%)	111/113 (98,2%)	118/135 (87,4%)	83/91 (91,2%)	94/95 (98,9%)	-
Cotrimoxazole (n/N')	54/54 (100%)	49/49 (100%)	59/141 (41,8%)	-	-	46/75 (61,3%)	72/95 (75,8%)	0,102
Rifampicin (n/N')	31/53 (58,5%)	10/48 (20,8%)	27/142 (19%)	67/113 (59,3%)	90/161 (55,9%)	16/90 (17,8%)	17/92 (18,5%)	0,029
Colistin (n/N')	0/54	0/51	0/142	0/107	0/157	0/79	0/4	-

n = number of resistant strains per year

N'= number of strains tested (this number varies according to the year and the antibiotic tested)

N= number of strains isolated per year

Table IV: Annual trends in antibiotic resistance in *P. aeruginosa*

	2010 (N=54)	2011 (N=101)	2012 (N=86)	2013 (N=72)	2014 (N=168)	2015 (N=81)	2016 (N=63)	P
Ticarcillin (n/N')	18/53 (34%)	38/101 (37,6%)	31/84 (36,9%)	33/72 (45,8%)	74/167 (44,3%)	21/67 (31,3%)	7/63 (11,1%)	0,058
Ticarcillin-Clavulanate (n/N')	17/54 (31,5%)	31/86 (36%)	25/66 (37,9%)	32/71 (45,1%)	68/149 (45,6%)	22/67 (32,8%)	7/63 (11,1%)	0,135
Piperacillin (n/N')	8/54 (14,8%)	36/101 (35,6%)	22/85 (25,9%)	19/66 (28,8%)	59/166 (35,5%)	12/40 (30%)	5/63 (7,9%)	0,408
Piperacillin-Tazobactam (n/N')	7/54 (13%)	36/100 (36%)	20/68 (29,4%)	18/71 (25,4%)	48/153 (31,4%)	12/39 (30,8%)	5/63 (7,9%)	0,218
Ceftazidime (n/N')	14/52 (26,9%)	35/101 (34,7%)	24/84 (28,6%)	19/72 (26,4%)	55/167 (32,9%)	14/67 (20,9%)	6/63 (9,5%)	**0,015**
Imipeneme (n/N')	14/53 (26,4%)	28/100 (28%)	20/86 (23,3%)	34/71 (47,9%)	76/168 (45,2%)	15/66 (22,7%)	13/63 (20,6%)	0,548
Amikacin (n/N')	9/54 (16,7%)	9/101 (8,9%)	13/86 (15,1%)	30/71 (42,3%)	51/167 (30,5%)	11/66 (16,7%)	2/62 (3,2%)	0,442
Ciprofloxacin (n/N')	14/54 (25,9%)	33/101 (32,7%)	43/86 (50%)	43/72 (59,7%)	91/147 (61,9%)	29/67 (43,3%)	5/63 (7,9%)	0,846
Cotrimoxazole (n/N')	49/53 (92,5%)	87/97 (89,7%)	75/84 (89,3%)	-	-	48/59 (81,4%)	-	-
Rifampicin (n/N')	50/50 (100%)	94/97 (96,9%)	76/80 (95%)	65/71 (91,5%)	142/166 (85,5%)	51/57 (89,5%)	-	-
Fosfomycin (n/N')	7/53 (13,2%)	16/98 (16,3%)	18/81 (22,2%)	68/72 (94,4%)	159/165 (96,4%)	8/40 (20%)	4/63 (6,3%)	**<0,001**
Colistin (n/N')	0/51	0/99	0/84	0/72	0/168	0/41	-	

n = number of resistant strains per year

N'= number of strains tested (this number varies according to the year and the antibiotic tested)

N= number of strains isolated per year

Table V: Annual trends in antibiotic resistance in *S. aureus*

	2010 (N=27)	2011 (N=52)	2012 (N=51)	2013 (N=34)	2014 (N=88)	2015 (N=83)	2016 (N=31)	P
Oxacillin (n/N')	3/27 (11,1%)	2/52 (3,8%)	1/51 (2%)	4/34 (11,8%)	11/88 (12,5%)	25/78 (32,1%)	6/30 (20%)	-
Amoxicillin (n/N')	26/27 (96,3%)	47/51 (92,2%)	48/51 (94,1%)	32/34 (94,1%)	71/88 (80,7%)	71/78 (91%)	29/30 (96,7%)	-
Kanamycin (n/N')	1/25 (4%)	13/52 (25%)	13/51 (25,5%)	6/34 (17,6%)	22/86 (25,6%)	30/78 (38,5%)	3/30 (10%)	0,1
Gentamicin (n/N')	1/26 (3,8%)	2/49 (4,1%)	0/51	3/33 (9,1%)	6/79 (7,6%)	22/78 (28,2%)	2/30 (6,7%)	-
Erythromycin (n/N')	1/27 (3,7%)	6/52 (11,5%)	4/51 (7,8%)	-	-	19/76 (25%)	3/30 (10%)	-
Lincomycin (n/N')	1/27 (3,7%)	2/52 (3,8%)	3/51 (5,9%)	4/34 (11,8%)	10/87 (11,5%)	9/76 (11,8%)	2/30 (6,7%)	-
Pristinamycin (n/N')	0/27	0/27	2/51 (3,9%)	0/34	11/88 (12,5%)	0/75	2/30 (6,7%)	-
Ofloxacin (n/N')	5/24 (20,8%)	2/50 (4%)	0/48	-	-	22/73 (30,1%)	4/30 (13,3%)	-
Vancomycin (n/N')	0/26	0/52	0/48	0/32	0/87	0/77	0/11	-
Teicoplanin (n/N')	0/26	0/52	0/47	0/34	0/88	0/75	0/11	-
Cotrimoxazole (n/N')	0/27	1/51 (2%)	0/50	-	-	4/74 (5,4%)	0/30	-
Fosfomycin (n/N')	1/26 (3,8%)	0/52	0/49	3/34 (8,8%)	3/88 (3,4%)	20/68 (29,4%)	1/30 (3,3%)	-
Rifampicin (n/N')	4/27 (14,8%)	2/52 (3,8%)	0/49	0/33	0/88	13/75 (17,3%)	2/30 (6,7%)	-
Fusidic acid (n/N')	2/14 (14,3%)	5/28 (17,9%)	3/27 (11,1%)	0/34	1/87 (1,1%)	3/49 (6,1%)	4/30 (13,3%)	-

n = number of resistant strains per year

N'= number of strains tested (this number varies according to the year and the antibiotic tested)

N= number of strains isolated per year

Table VI: Annual evolution of antibiotic resistance in *E.faecalis*

	2010 (N=19)	2011 (N=115)	2012 (N=152)	2013 (N=46)	2014 (N=48)	2015 (N=44)	2016 (N=52)	P
Amoxicillin (n/N')	0 /19	3/114 (2,6%)	2/152 (1,3%)	0/45	1/48 (2,1%)	1/42 (2,4%)	-	-
Kanamycin (n/N')	15/19 (78,9%)	66/114 (57,9%)	151/151 (100%)	1/46 (2,2%)	1/48 (2,1%)	22/35 (62,9%)	-	<0,001
Gentamicin (n/N')	3/19 (15,8%)	47/115 (40,9%)	151/151 (100%)	46/46 (100%)	47/47 (100%)	19/36 (52,8%)	-	-
Erythromycin (n/N')	16/18 (88,9%)	105/115 (91,3%)	132/146 (90,4%)	-	-	36/42 (85,7%)	41/49 (83,7%)	-
Pristinamycin (n/N')	15/18 (83,3%)	112/114 (98,2%)	111/144 (77,1%)	-	-	27/36 (75%)	28/47 (59,6%)	-
Levofloxacin (n/N')	2/3 (66,7%)	6/15 (40%)	1/18 (5,6%)	-	-	1/18 (5,6%)	0/49	-
Vancomycin (n/N')	0/18	1/114 (0,9%)	0/145	-	-	0/41	0/49	-
Teicoplanin (n/N')	0/18	0/114	0/145	1/46 (2,2%)	1/48 (2,1%)	0/42	0/48	-
Cotrimoxazole (n/N')	19/19 (100%)	112/113 (99,1%)	85/144 (59%)	-	-	22/40 (55%)	49/49 (100%)	-
Fosfomycin (n/N')	17/17 (100%)	112/114 (98,2%)	151/151 (100%)	4/42 (9,5%)	9/48 (18,8%)	33/34 (97,1%)	1/48 (2,1%)	-
Rifampicin (n/N')	1/19 (5,3%)	10/110 (9,1%)	8/92 (8,7%)	37/46 (80,4%)	31/48 (64,6%)	2/32 (6,3%)	30/49 (61,2%)	<0,001

n = number of resistant strains per year

N'= number of strains tested (this number varies according to the year and the antibiotic tested)

N= number of strains isolated per year

Annual evolution of BMR in the four services concerned:

The annual evolution of the 9 BMR monitored at Sahloul hospital, namely cefotaxime-resistant *K. pneumoniae* (*K. pneumoniae* CTX-R), cefotaxime-resistant *E. coli (E. coli* CTX-R), ertapenem-resistant *K. pneumoniae* (*K. pneumoniae* ETP-R), ertapenem-resistant *E. coli* (*E. coli* ETP-R), imipenem-resistant *A. baumannii (A. baumannii* IMP-R), ceftazidime-resistant *P. aeruginosa* (*P. aeruginosa* CAZ-R), imipenem-resistant *P. aeruginosa* (*P. aeruginosa* IMP-R), methicillin-resistant *S. aureus* (MRSA), and glycopeptide-resistant enterococci (GRE), is reported in Figure 5

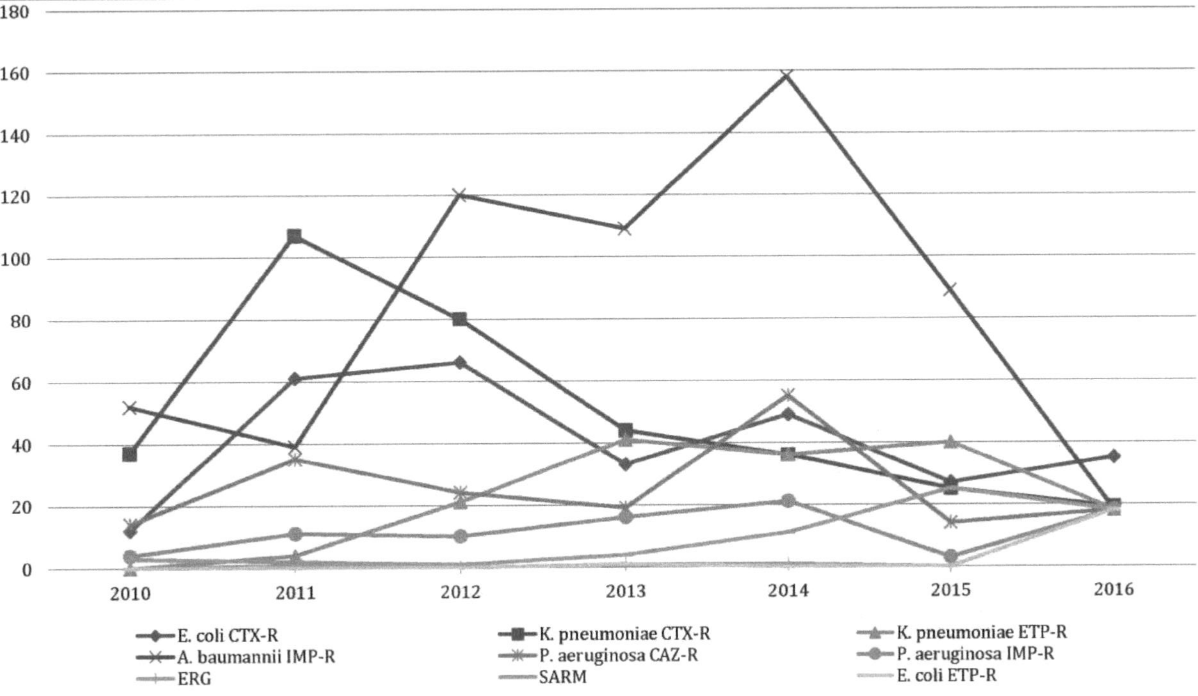

Figure 5: Overall annual change in BMRs

Department of Urology:

Samples :

The specimens from the urology department were urocultures (n=2246, 84.7%), deep suppurations (n=191, 7.2%) and blood cultures (n=179, 6.8%) (**Figure 6**).

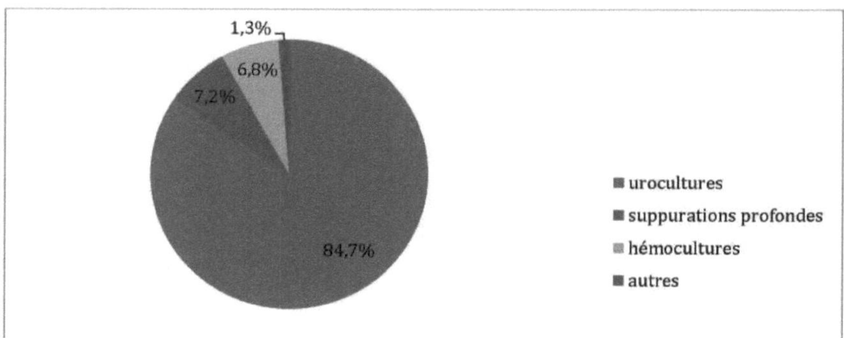

Figure 6: Samples taken in the urology department

Isolated germs :

A total of 2651 strains were isolated from the urology department: *E. coli* (n=1068, 40.3%), *K. pneumoniae* (n=479, 18.1%), *E. faecalis* (n=341, 12.9%), *E. cloacae* (n=129, 4.9%), *P. aeruginosa* (n=98, 3.7%), and Group B Streptococcus (n=85, 3.2%) (**Figure 7**).

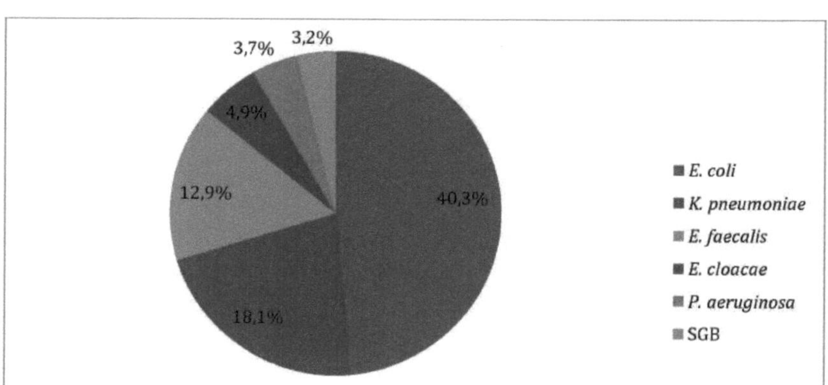

Figure 7: Bacteria isolated in the urology department

The results of the stratification of the germs isolated in the urology department according to the samples are reported in table VII.

Table VII: Distribution of germs according to the samples taken in the urology department:

	E. coli	*K. pneumoniae*	*E. faecalis*	*E. cloacae*	*P. aeruginosa*	*S. agalactiae*
ECBU	935 (41,6%)	414 (18,4%)	309 (13,8%)	116 (5,2%)	81 (3,6%)	80 (3,6%)
Blood cultures	67 (37,4%)	47 (26,3%)	13 (7,3%)	7 (3,9%)	3 (1,7%)	1 (0,6%)
Deeper	53 (27,7%)	15 (7,9%)	18 (9,4%)	5 (2,6%)	11 (5,8%)	5 (2,6%)

Resistance profile of isolated bacteria to antibiotics :

Antibiotic resistance patterns of the main bacteria isolated in the urology department are described in Tables VIII to X.

The annual evolution of BMR isolated in the urology department is reported in figure 8.

Table VIII: Resistance profile of the most frequently isolated enterobacteria in the urology department:

	E. coli	*K. pneumoniae*	*E. cloacae*
Amoxicillin	743 (69,8%)	474 (99,8%)	-
Amoxicillin-Clavulanate	481 (45,2%)	340 (71,6%)	-
Cephalotin	333 (33,2%)	249 (55,6%)	-
Cefotaxime	227 (21,4%)	224 (51,4%)	78 (60,5%)
Cefoxitin	32 (3%)	42 (8,9%)	-
Imipenem	0	22 (4,6%)	1 (0,8%)
Ertapenem	2 (0,2%)	35 (7,4%)	4 (3,1%)
Gentamicin	215 (20,2%)	201 (42,7%)	47 (36,4%)
Amikacin	4 (0,4%)	74 (15,6%)	6 (4,7%)
Nalidixic acid	422 (46,9%)	229 (58,7%)	46 (42,2%)
Ofloxacin	444 (48,6%)	233 (61,5%)	50 (45%)
Ciprofloxacin	520 (49%)	298 (63,3%)	62 (48,1%)
Cotrimoxazole	465 (51,3%)	163 (43,2%)	40 (36%)
Fosfomycin	4 (0,4%)	11 (3%)	6 (5,5%)
Chloramphenicol	35 (12,3%)	21 (15,1%)	5 (19,2%)
Colistin	0	1 (0,2%)	0
Nitrofurantoin	19 (2,6%)	100 (32,1%)	52 (53,6%)

Table IX: Resistance profile of *Pseudomonas aeruginosa* strains isolated from the urology department:

Antibiotic	N	%
Ticarcillin	45	53
Piperacillin	38	40,4
Piperacillin-Tazobactam	36	41,4
Ceftazidime	39	40,6
Imipenem	10	10,3
Gentamicin	14	14,3
Amikacin	10	10,2
Ciprofloxacin	60	61,2
Fosfomycin	19	21,3
Rifampicin	79	94
Colistin	0	0

Table X: Antibiotic resistance profile of *E. faecalis* and group B streptococci strains isolated in the urology department:

	E. faecalis	Streptococcus group B
Ampicillin	5 (1,6%)	0
Ampicillin-Clavulanate	3 (1,1%)	0
Teicoplanin	1 (0,3%)	0
Vancomycin	1 (0,3%)	0
Gentamicin (NHN)	234 (76,5%)	48 (57,1%)
Erythromycin	258 (89,9%)	22 (26,8%)
Lincomycin	329 (98,2%)	22 (25,6%)
Pristinamycin	234 (83,3%)	2 (2,5%)
Levofloxacin	1 (4,2%)	0
Moxifloxacin	47 (2,1%)	-
Nitrofurantoin	49 (19,8%)	4 (6,2%)
Rifampicin	66 (24,1%)	6 (9,4%)
Cotrimoxazole	220 (78%)	2 (2,5%)

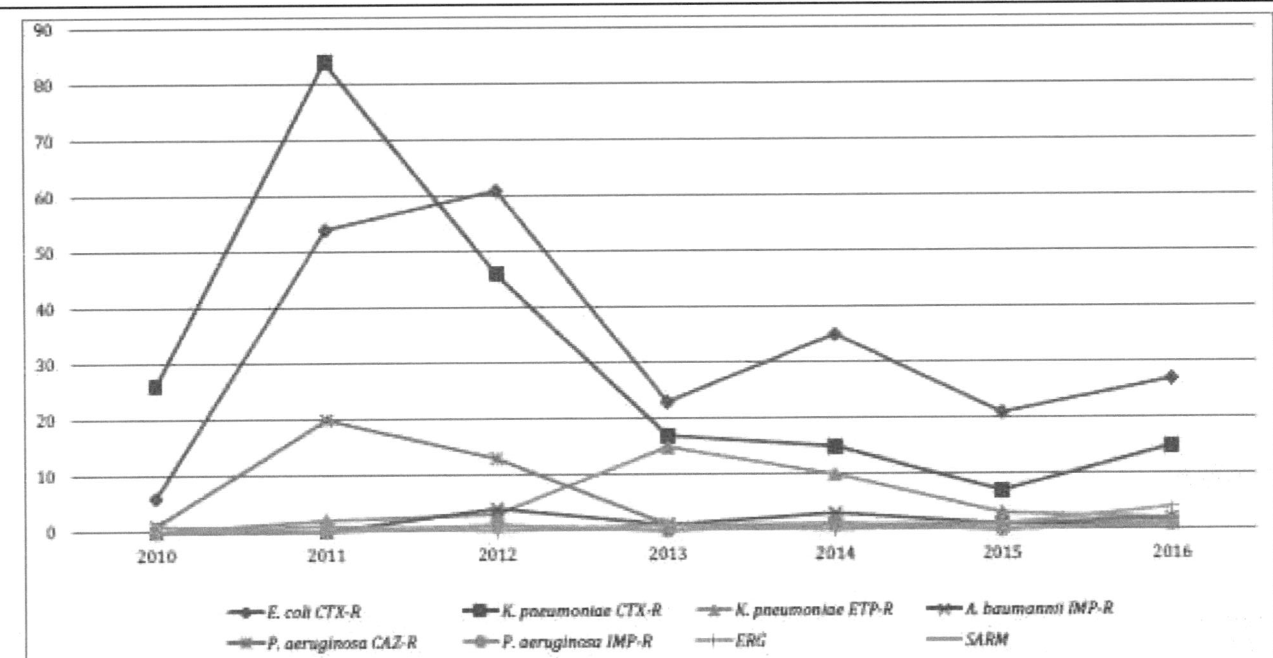

Figure 8: Annual evolution of BMR in urology

POG Service:

Samples :

Bacteriological samples taken in the POG department were blood cultures (35.4%), ECBU (17.2%), medical devices (15.9%) and protected distal samples (14.5%) **(Figure 9)**.

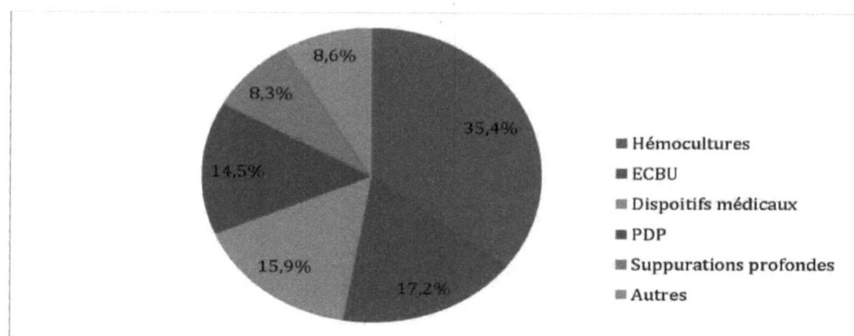

Figure 9: Samples taken at POG

Isolated germs :

A. baumannii, K. pneumoniae, P. aeruginosa and *S. aureus* were isolated in 21.5%, 15.6%, 14.7% and 10.4% of cases respectively **(Figure 10)**.

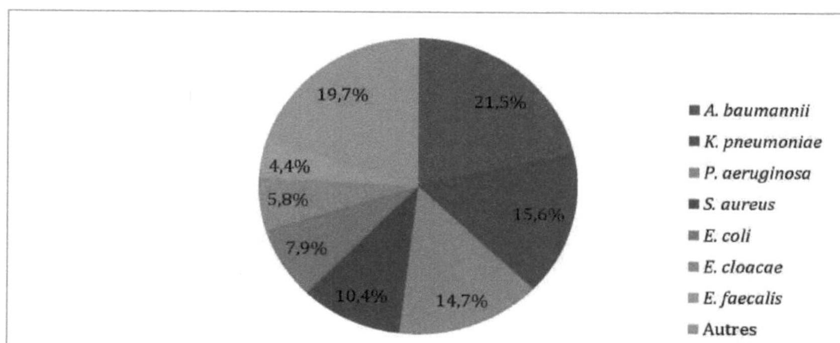

Figure 10: Bacteria isolated in the POG department

The distribution of the germs isolated in the POG department according to the samples is reported in table XI.

Table XI: Distribution of germs isolated in the POG department according to the samples :

	A. baumannii	K. pneumoniae	P. aeruginosa	S. aureus	E. coli	E. cloacae	E. faecalis
Blood	13 (26,8%	111 (22,6%	4 (8,7%)	40 (8,1%)	23 (4,7%)	48 (9,8%	18 (3,7%)
ECBU	4 (17,6%	4 (18,4%	2 (10,9%	2 (0,8%)	44 (18,4%)	9 (3,8%	23 (9,6%)
Devices medical	5 (26,2%	2 (13,1%	5 (23,1%	24 (10,9%)	17 (7,7%)	10 (4,5%	7 (3,2%
PDP	37 (18,4%	129 (6%)	3 (19,4%	59 (29,4%)	5 (2,5%)	2 (1%)	3 (1,5%)
Deeper	1 (11,3%	8 (7%)	1 (16,5%	7 (6,1%)	12 (10,4%)	4 (3,5%	5 (4,3%)

Resistance profile of bacteria isolated to antibiotics in the POG department:

The bacterial resistances of the main species isolated in the POG department are described in Tables XII to XIV.

The annual evolution of the BMRs monitored in the urology department is reported in figure 11.

Table XII: Antibiotic resistance profile of non-fermentative BGN in the POG department:

	A. baumannii	P. aeruginosa
Ticarcillin	257 (96,3%)	40 (20,4%)
Ticarcillin-Clavulanate	245 (96,1%)	38 (20%)
Piperacillin	203 (96,2%)	36 (18,9%)
Piperacillin-T azobactam	196 (95,6%)	32 (17,7%)
Ceftazidime	187 (87,8%)	32 (16,2%)
Imipeneme	253 (94,4%)	58 (29,3%)
Amikacin	237 (88,8%)	26 (13,2%)
Ciprofloxacin	232 (89,9%)	49 (25,4%)
Cotrimoxazole	103 (68,2%)	82 (82,8%)
Fosfomycin	-	84 (44,7%)
Rifampicin	94 (35,7%)	143 (86,1%)
Chloramphenicol	196 (99,5%)	-
Colistin	0	0

Table XIII: Antibiotic resistance profile of Enterobacteriaceae in the POG department:

	K. pneumoniae	*E. coli*	*E. cloacae*
Amoxicillin	-	89 (84%)	-
Amoxicillin-Clavulanate	128 (61,2%)	44 (41,9%)	-
Cefoxitin	27 (15,4%)	7 (7,6%)	-
Cefotaxime	79 (38%)	12 (11,3%)	38 (48,7%)
Ertapenem	36 (18,7%)	0	3 (4,7%)
Imipenem	22 (10,5%)	0	0
Nalidixic acid	24 (43,6%)	12 (28,6%)	10 (47,6%)
Ofloxacin	55 (43,3%)	25 (36,2%)	16 (28,1%)
Ciprofloxacin	90 (43,5%)	30 (29,1%)	18 (23,4%)
Gentamicin	81 (39,1%)	19 (18,3%)	21 (27,3%)
Amikacin	30 (14,4%)	2 (1,9%)	3 (3,8%)
Cotrimoxazole	48 (40%)	38 (57,6%)	16 (28,6%)
Fosfomycin	7 (6 ,1%)	0	3 (5,7%)
Rifampicin	37 (45,7%)	22 (59,5%)	6 (28,6%)
Chloramphenicol	24 (13,3%)	13 (17,1%)	21 (29,6%)
Colistin	1 (0,6%)	0	0

Table XIV: Antibiotic resistance profile of Gram-positive cocci isolated in the POG department:

	S. aureus	*E. faecalis*
Oxacillin	21 (14,7%)	-
Amoxicillin	128 (89,5%)	1 (2,2%)
Kanamycin	33 (23,2%)	16 (34,8%)
Gentamicin	13 (9,5%)	35 (76,1%)
Erythromycin	13 (13,8%)	30 (83,3%)
Lincomycin	13 (9,2%)	-
Pristinamycin	12 (8,5%)	22 (71%)
Ofloxacin	9 (10%)	-
Levofloxacin	-	3 (13,6%)
Vancomycin	0	0
Teicoplanin	0	1 (1,8%)
Cotrimoxazole	2 (2,2%)	28 (80%)
Fosfomycin	9 (6,7%)	30 (52,6%)
Rifampicin	7 (5%)	28 (51,9%)
Fusidic acid	4 (3,6%)	-

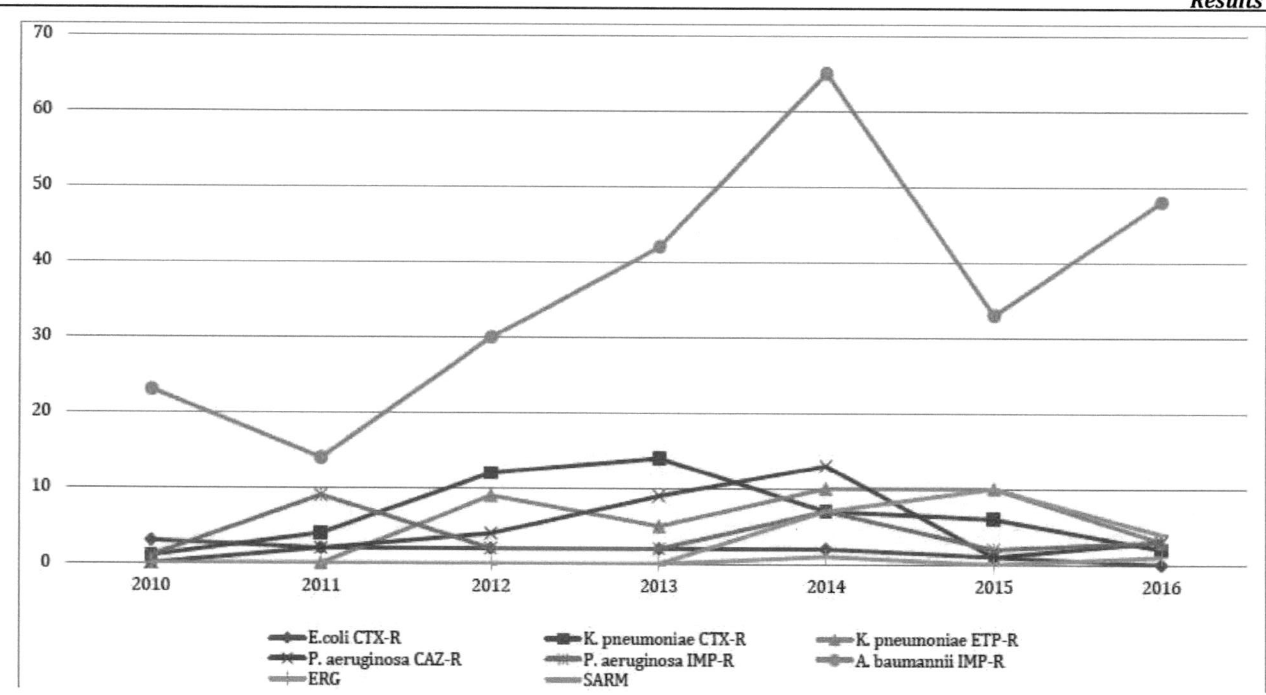

Figure 11: Annual evolution of BMRs in the POG department

Surgical Resuscitation Service :
Samples :

The samples taken in the surgical resuscitation unit were blood cultures, protected distal samples, medical devices and UECs in 34.8%, 17%, 15.7% and 14.3% of cases respectively **(Figure 12)**.

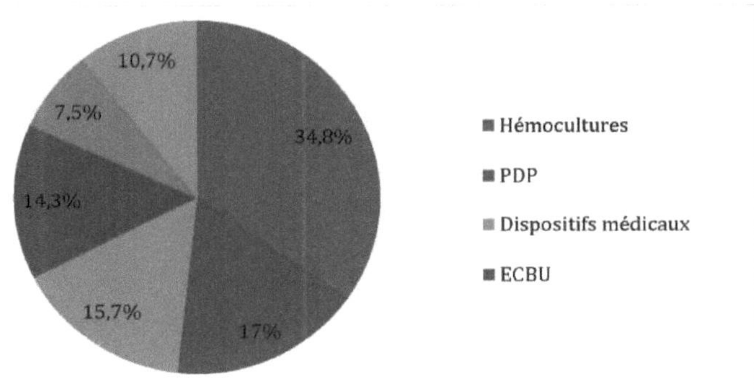

Figure 12: Samples taken in the Surgical Intensive Care Unit

Isolated germs :

Non-fermentative BGN were isolated in 20.8% of cases for *A. baumannii* and 15.3% of cases for *P. aeruginosa* **(Figure 13)**.

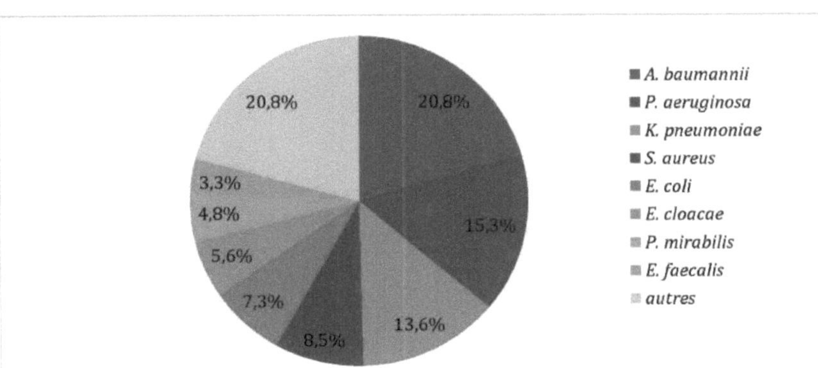

Figure 13: Bacteria isolated from the surgical resuscitation unit

The distribution of the most frequently isolated bacteria in the surgical resuscitation unit is described in Table XV.

Table XV: Distribution of germs isolated in the surgical resuscitation department according to the samples :

	A. baumannii	P. aeruginosa	K. pneumoniae	S. aureus	E. coli	E. cloacae	P. mirabilis	E. faecalis
Blood cultures	124 (21,6%)	61 (10,6%)	104 (18,1%)	22 (3,8%)	21 (3,7%)	47 (8,2%)	32 (5,6%)	20 (3,5%)
PDP	49 (17,4%)	54 (19,2%)	23 (8,2%)	82 (29,2%)	10 (3,6%)	9 (3,2%)	4 (1,4%)	2 (0,7%)
Medical devices	79 (30,5%)	60 (23,2%)	32 (12,4%)	12 (4,6%)	13 (5%)	13 (5%)	5 (1,9%)	2 (0,8%)
ECBU	43 (18,2%)	31 (13,1%)	41 (17,4%)	0	56 (23,7%)	8 (3,4%)	15 (6,4%)	17 (7,2%)
Deeper	14 (11,3%)	15 (12,1%)	10 (8,1%)	6 (4,8%)	11 (8,9%)	5 (4%)	11 (8,9%)	6 (4,8%)

Resistance profile of bacteria isolated to antibiotics in the surgical resuscitation unit:

Resistance patterns of the major bacterial species isolated from the surgical resuscitation unit are reported in Tables XVI to XVIII.

The annual evolution of the BMRs monitored in the surgical resuscitation department is described in figure 14.

Table XVI: Antibiotic resistance profile of non-fermentative BGN in the surgical resuscitation unit :

	A. baumannii	*P. aeruginosa*
Ticarcillin	320 (98,8%)	99 (40,7%)
Ticarcillin-Clavulanate	302 (99%)	92 (40,9%)
Piperacillin	276 (98,6%)	55 (23,9%)
Piperacillin-T azobactam	260 (97,7%)	52 (23,2%)
Ceftazidime	272 (94,4%)	63 (25,9%)
Imipeneme	315 (96,6%)	95 (39,3%)
Amikacin	295 (91%)	62 (25,6%)
Ciprofloxacin	296 (95,5%)	103 (44,4%)
Cotrimoxazole	126 (65,6%)	85 (80,2%)
Fosfomycin	-	127 (55,5%)
Rifampicin	110 (34,5%)	197 (92,9%)
Colistin	0	0

Table XVII: Antibiotic resistance profile of Enterobacteriaceae in the surgical resuscitation unit :

	K. pneumoniae	*E. coli*	*E. cloacae*	*P. mirabilis*
Amoxicillin	-	90 (79,6%)	-	66 (83,5%)
Amoxicillin-Clavulanate	168 (77,4%)	55 (48,7%)	-	48 (60,8%)
Cefoxitin	63 (34,2%)	6 (6,3%)	-	24 (33,8)
Cefotaxime	132 (61,1%)	37 (32,7%)	43 (49,4%)	45 (58,4%)
Ertapenem	62 (30,8%)	0	7 (9,1%)	1 (1,4%)
Imipenem	44 (20,3%)	0	2 (2,3%)	1 (1,3%)
Nalidixic acid	49 (62%)	12 (29,3%)	4 (23,5%)	3 (37,5%)
Ofloxacin	86 (64,2%)	25 (35,7%)	9 (15,8%)	11 (23,4%)
Ciprofloxacin	135 (62,2%)	44 (40,4%)	19 (22,6%)	17 (23,3%)
Gentamicin	119 (55,9%)	27 (25%)	17 (19,8%)	28 (36,8%)
Amikacin	51 (23,6%)	10 (9%)	1 (1,1%)	37 (46,8%)
Cotrimoxazole	74 (57,4%)	34 (50,7%)	10 (18,9%)	30 (68,2%)
Fosfomycin	9 (7%)	0	0	11 (24,4%)
Rifampicin	33 (40,2%)	27 (62,8%)	10 (32,3%)	16 (50%)
Chloramphenicol	51 (26,8%)	12 (17,1%)	20 (26,3%)	25 (40,3%)
Colistin	1 (0,5%)	0	0	-

Table XVIII: Antibiotic resistance profile of Gram-positive cocci isolated from the surgical resuscitation unit :

	S. aureus	*E. faecalis*
Oxacillin	24 (17,5%)	-
Amoxicillin	125 (91,9%)	1 (2,2%)
Kanamycin	36 (26,5%)	16 (36,4%)
Gentamicin	20 (15,3%)	33 (73,3%)
Erythromycin	11 (12,8%)	30 (88,2%)
Lincomycin	10 (7,3%)	-
Pristinamycin	2 (1,5%)	25 (73,5%)
Ofloxacin	20 (24,4%)	-
Levofloxacin	-	3 (12,5%)
Vancomycin	0	0
Teicoplanin	0	0
Cotrimoxazole	2 (2,4%)	27 (77,1%)
Fosfomycin	15 (11,1%)	30 (58,8%)
Rifampicin	12 (8,8%)	18 (36,7%)
Fusidic acid	7 (7,7%)	-

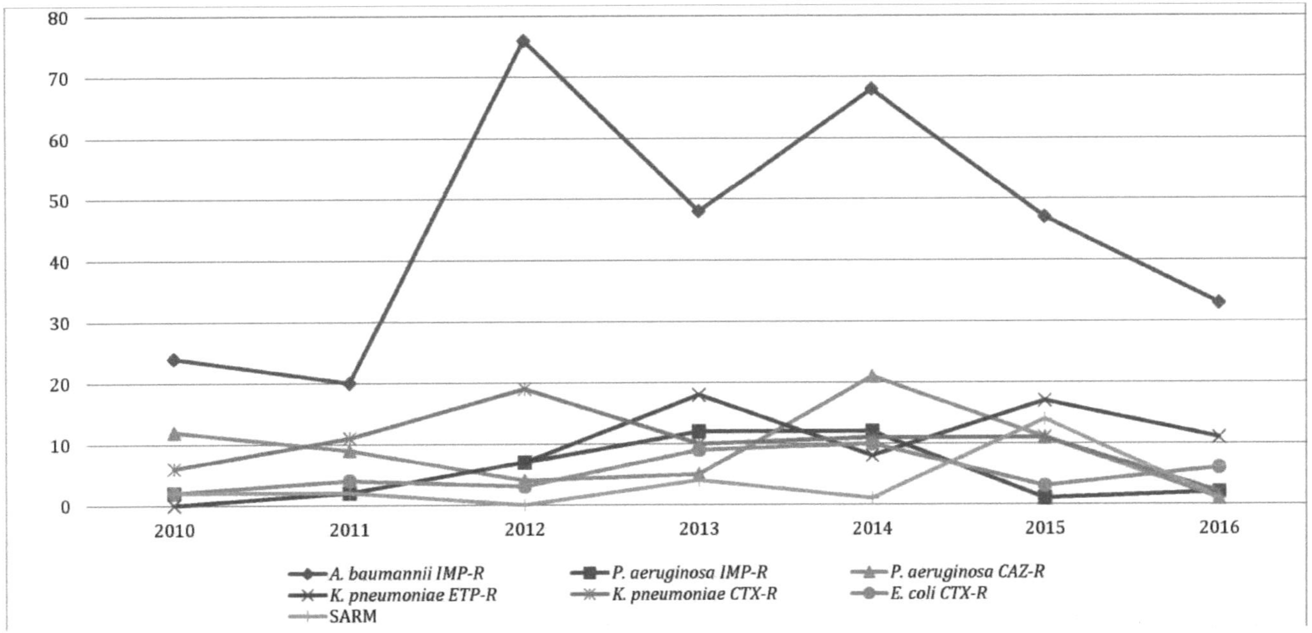

Figure 14: Annual evolution of BMR in the surgical resuscitation department

Medical Resuscitation Service :

Samples :

Blood cultures, ECBU and protected distal swabs were performed in 28.9%, 18.4% and 15% of cases respectively (**Figure 15**).

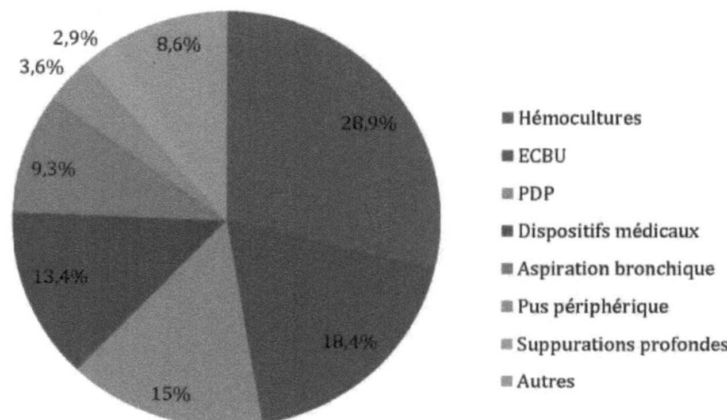

Figure 15: samples taken in the medical intensive care unit

Isolated germs :

The germs isolated in the medical intensive care unit were *A. baumannii, K. pneumoniae* **and** *P. aeruginosa* in 20.8%, 17.2% and 16.7% of cases respectively (**Figure 16**).

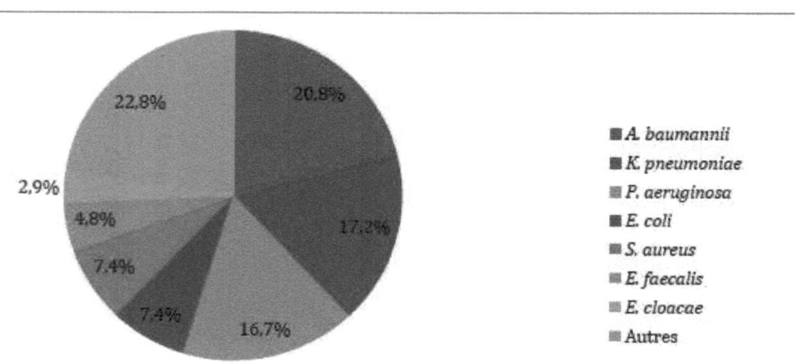

Figure 16: Germs isolated in the medical intensive care unit

The distribution of the main germs isolated in the medical resuscitation department according to the samples is presented in table XIX.

Table XIX: Distribution of germs isolated in the medical intensive care unit according to the samples :

	A. baumannii	K. pneumoniae	P. aeruginosa	E. coli	S. aureus	E. faecalis	E. cloacae
Blood cultures	30 (24,8%)	29 (24%)	7 (5,8%)	2 (1,7%)	4 (3,3%)	5 (4,1%)	9 (7,4%)
ECBU	5 (6,5%)	13 (16,9%)	19 (24,7%)	19 (24,7%)	0	9 (11,7%)	0
PDP	12 (19%)	4 (6,3%)	12 (19%)	1 (1,6%)	11 (17,5%)	2 (3,2%)	0
Medical devices	16 (28,6%)	15 (26,8%)	8 (14,3%)	6 (10,7%)	0	2 (3,6%)	3 (5,4%)
Bronchial suction	13 (33,3%)	4 (10,3%)	8 (20,5%)	0	6 (15,4%)	1 (2,6%)	0
More peripheral	3 (20%)	2 (13,3%)	4 (26,7%)	1 (6,7%)	1 (6,7%)	0	0
Deep Suppurations	1 (8,3%)	3 (25%)	5 (41,7%)	0	0	1 (8,3%)	0

Resistance profile of bacteria isolated to antibiotics in the medical intensive care unit:

The resistance profiles of the main bacteria isolated in the medical intensive care unit are reported in Tables XX to XXII.

The annual evolution of the BMRs monitored in the medical intensive care unit is described in figure 17.

Table XX: Antibiotic resistance profile of non-fermentative BGN in the medical intensive care unit :

	A. baumannii	*P. aeruginosa*
Ticarcillin	84 (100%)	38 (54,3%)
Ticarcillin-Clavulanate	76 (100%)	37 (56,1%)
Piperacillin	69 (98,6%)	32 (51,6%)
Piperacillin-Tazobactam	66 (98,5%)	26 (46,4%)
Ceftazidime	64 (88,9%)	33 (47,1%)
Imipeneme	82 (96,5%)	37 (52,9%)
Amikacin	73 (88%)	27 (38,6%)
Ciprofloxacin	76 (98,7%)	46 (68,7%)
Cotrimoxazole	34 (82,9%)	24 (85,7%)
Fosfomycin	-	50 (75,8%)
Rifampicin	48 (57,8%)	59 (96,7%)
Chloramphenicol	65 (100%)	-
Colistin	0	0

Table XXI: Antibiotic resistance profile of Enterobacteriaceae isolated in the medical intensive care unit :

	K. pneumoniae	*E. coli*	*E. cloacae*
Amoxicillin	-	22 (71%)	-
Amoxicillin-Clavulanate	59 (85,5%)	13 (41,9%)	-
Cefoxitin	22 (35,5%)	4 (13,8%)	-
Cefotaxime	47 (68,1%)	9 (29%)	9 (81,8%)
Ertapenem	25 (41,7%)	0	1 (10%)
Imipenem	15 (21,7%)	0	0
Nalidixic acid	20 (76,9%)	9 (60%)	2 (100%)
Ofloxacin	32 (68,1%)	11 (55%)	7 (87,5%)
Ciprofloxacin	48 (70,6%)	14 (45,2%)	10 (90,9%)
Gentamicin	35 (51,5%)	5 (16,1%)	7 (63,6%)
Amikacin	23 (33,3%)	4 (12,9%)	3 (27,3%)
Cotrimoxazole	19 (40,9%)	15 (75%)	8 (100%)
Fosfomycin	12 (27,3%)	0	0
Rifampicin	10 (45,5%)	4 (36,4%)	3 (100%)
Chloramphenicol	21 (36,8%)	4 (20%)	4 (40%)
Colistin	3 (4,8%)	0	0

Table XXII: Antibiotic resistance profile of gram-positive cocci isolated in the medical intensive care unit :

	S. aureus	*E. faecalis*
Oxacillin	3 (10%)	-
Amoxicillin	29 (96,7%)	0
Kanamycin	10 (33,3%)	7 (41,2%)
Gentamicin	2 (6,7%)	11 (64,7%)
Erythromycin	2 (10%)	12 (92,3%)
Lincomycin	3 (10%)	-
Pristinamycin	2 (1,5%)	25 (73,5%)
Ofloxacin	1 (5%)	-
Levofloxacin	-	3 (37,5%)
Vancomycin	0	0
Teicoplanin	0	0
Cotrimoxazole	1 (4,8%)	12 (92,3%)
Fosfomycin	2 (6,9%)	12 (63,2%)
Rifampicin	1 (3,6%)	7 (36,8%)
Fusidic acid	3 (15%)	-

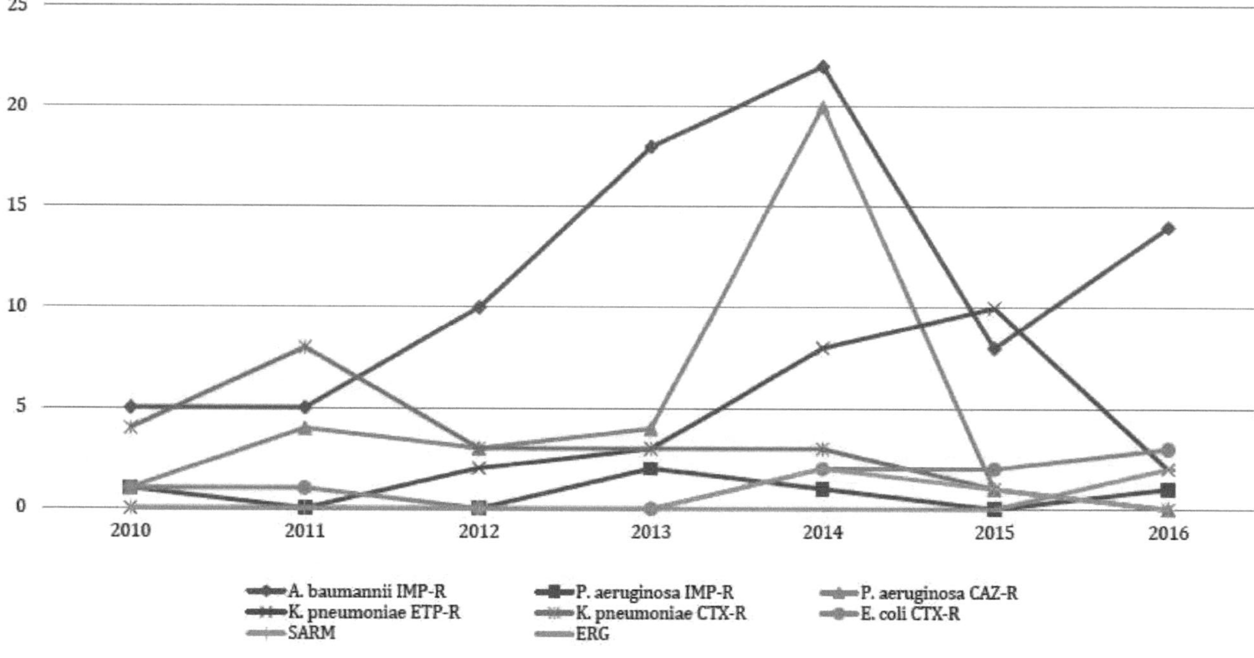

Figure 17: Annual evolution of BMR in the medical intensive care unit

Discussion

Discussion:

Bacterial resistance to antibiotics is the main cause of therapeutic failure in the treatment of infections. This phenomenon found in the city and especially in hospitals is the daily concern of the microbiology laboratory, whose mission is to monitor the evolution of antibiotic resistance of bacteria involved in clinical trials and thus identify the bacterial ecology of the various hospital services in order to guide antibiotic therapy, which is often probabilistic at first and then adapted to the microbiological results at a later stage.

This is the context of our work, which completes an epidemiological study conducted in our hospital from 2001 to 2005 and which identified the urology, POG, surgical resuscitation and medical resuscitation departments as being those at high risk of BMR infection(14). This guided our focus on these four departments to describe the evolution of antibiotic resistance in our hospital.

Discussion of the methodology :

This is a retrospective study carried out within the framework of the microbiology laboratory's surveillance of bacterial resistance to antibiotics. This method, which is based on the collection and analysis of data available in the laboratory computerization system, is used by several national and international networks responsible for the surveillance of antibiotic resistance, for example LART in Tunisia, ONERBA in France and ECDC in Europe.

The advantage of this retrospective passive surveillance is that it is simple, inexpensive and gives an idea of the bacterial ecology of the clinical services concerned. On the other hand, it also has some disadvantages.

Without access to clinical records, the isolation of a bacterium from a specimen does not always mean that it is responsible for the infection, except for certain biological products, such as cerebrospinal fluid or serous fluids, where interpretation is easier.

In addition, this passive surveillance only provides information on strains isolated routinely. Active surveillance of certain infections, such as community-acquired infections, must be done prospectively since the indications for microbiological sampling are generally limited (22).

Due to the annual change in the CA-SFM and then CA-SFM/EUCAST recommendations, the search for antibiotic resistance was not performed in the same way for the entire study period, so there may be some bias in the interpretation of the susceptibility of some bacteria to antibiotics.

Sometimes an interpretative reading was recommended, as was the case in 2013 when the laboratory returned a susceptible or intermediate resistant result for penicillins and third generation cephalosporins in the case of ESBL-producing enterobacteria. This recommendation was changed in subsequent years and the laboratory would then report the raw result without an interpretative reading. This could have overestimated the rate of resistance found in 2013 (18,19).

Despite the limitations reported above, this method of passive surveillance remains necessary because it allows the microbiology laboratory to play an essential role in guiding clinical services in the choice of probabilistic treatments, orienting the policy of antibiotic use within a health care institution or at the level of a population, and thus contributing to the hygiene policy (22).

The simplicity of this method also allows microbiology laboratories, in hospitals or in towns, to easily join national or international surveillance networks, subject to standardised working methods, and thus to increase the collective database, which will help to guide health authorities in establishing priority areas for action in terms of bacterial resistance to antibiotics. These data collected will also allow the learned societies to update their recommendations in the management of infections according to the local reality.

During the seven years of the study, the most frequently isolated germs were Enterobacteriaceae with *E. coli* as the leader followed by *K. pneumoniae. The* next most frequent isolates were non-fermenting Gram-negative bacilli: *A. baumannii* and *P. aeruginosa.* Gram-positive cocci are in [third] place and are represented mainly by *E. faecalis* and *S. aureus* with less than 8% of isolates each. These germs came mainly from cytobacteriological examinations of urine, blood cultures, medical devices and protected distal samples. In terms of departmental distribution, enterobacteriaceae were the most frequent organisms in the urology department and non-fermenting gram-negative bacilli, especially *A. baumannii*, were the most frequent organisms in the three intensive care units. Gram-negative bacilli have overtaken gram-positive cocci in terms of nosocomial infections in recent years, and particularly ESBL-producing Enterobacteriaceae, which have taken the lead ahead of MRSA, which has tended to decrease in the hospital setting (23). Until the 2000s, staphylococci were the leading bacteria responsible for nosocomial infections; in neonatology, coagulase-negative staphylococci were the first germs incriminated in intensive care units (24). There was then a change in bacterial epidemiology, in fact, several national and international studies affirm that the role of staphylococcus and MRSA in particular has regressed to the benefit of Gram-negative bacilli. In a symposium on "Current Aspects of Emerging Multidrug Resistant Bacteria" in 2012 in Paris, J. C Lucet announced that data from the surveillance network of 312 French health care institutions confirm that MRSA are no longer at the forefront of resistant bacteria and have been replaced by E-BLSE (25). A Moroccan study published in 2014 reports that the predominant germs in a neonatal intensive care unit are enterobacteria (26) and a Tunisian study published the same year confirms that the most multidrug-resistant bacteria isolated in the neonatology unit of Monastir are enterobacteria resistant to third-generation cephalosporins (27).

Escherichia coli

Escherichia coli is the most frequent germ in our series given the particularities of our population; the urology department being the first department requesting urocultures but also the one where we found the most isolates. From a global point of view, _E. coli_ is the first germ isolated in the microbiology laboratories of the different Tunisian or international hospitals (10,28).

This group 1 enterobacterium is naturally sensitive to beta-lactams. However, it produces a very low level of a non-inducible chromosomal cephalosporinase of the AmpC type (29). We identified a wild type phenotype in 30.2% of cases in the urology department and in 15 to 30% of cases in the three intensive care units. This resistance to aminopenicillins is restored by beta-lactamase inhibitors but the prevalence of resistance to the combination of amoxicillin and clavulanic acid remains high (about 40 to 50%). We have noticed an overall trend of increasing resistance to cefotaxime, fluoroquinolones and gentamicin. On the other hand, resistance to amikacin seems to remain stable.

Resistance to cefotaxime has rapidly increased from 12.8% in 2010 to 38.7% in 2016. This is explained by the acquisition of other resistance mechanisms in E. coli strains, mainly extended-spectrum beta-lactamases (ESBL). These enzymes confer resistance to penicillins and cephalosporins to varying degrees in the enterobacteria that produce them, with the exception of cephamycins. Carbapenems remain active on these strains (29). Antibiograms performed according to the recommendations of the CA- SFM/EUCAST allow phenotypic identification of ESBLs by qualitative or quantitative methods.

At the molecular level, ESBLs are the source of mutated class A transferable beta-lactamases (TEM/SHV) with increased affinity for various beta-lactams including C3Gs. Other transferable enzymes such as CTX-M and MEN-1(30) soon appeared. Today, there are more than 150 described types of ESBLs in the world. Depending on the type of enzyme, there will be preferential hydrolysis of cefotaxime or ceftazidime (31). CTX-M, whose preferential substrate is cefotaxime, has very quickly taken the lead in E-BLSE in our country and in the world; indeed, a study carried out on clinical strains of _E. coli_ at the Military Hospital and the Habib Thameur Hospital in Tunis identified the plasmid gene _blaCTX-M15_ for all isolates (32). This same result is supported by a study performed on Palestinian clinical _E. coli_ strains which identified _blaerX-M15_ as the first ESBL coding gene among the isolates studied (33). A study conducted in our laboratory also showed that ESBL-producing Enterobacteriaceae isolated from patients hospitalized in the urology and intensive care units carried CTX-M15-encoding genes in 91% of cases (34). Mnif et al. also reported that 72.4% of _E. coli_ ESBL strains carried the _blaCTX-M_ gene and 62% carried the _blaCTX-M-15 gene_ (35).

In our series, we found a significant association between resistance to third-generation cephalosporins and resistance to fluoroquinolones and aminoglycosides. This has also been found in other studies and may be explained by the plasmid determinism of resistance to these three classes of antibiotics (36,37).

Several risk factors for EBLSE infection have been identified in the literature, such as age >=65 years, female gender, healthcare-associated bacteremia, cirrhosis, obstructive uropathy, urinary catheterization, recent antibiotic therapy, long hospital stay, and use of fluoroquinolones (38). The presence of resistance genes in the environment and in food animals also appear to be risk factors for transmission of ESBL strains to humans (39,40).

Carbapenem resistance is still very rare in *E. coli* in our series (1.1% resistance to ertapenem in 2016 and no resistance to imipenem). In 2014, LART data reported 0.2% resistance to imipenem (10). In an Indian study, the prevalence of *E. coli* strain resistance to imipenem was 10% by production of NDM-type carbapenemase (41). There is therefore a real risk of diffusion of carbapenemases in *E. coli,* which should alert us to implement preventive measures to delay the appearance of this phenomenon as much as possible.

K. pneumoniae

K. pneumoniae is the second most frequently found enterobacterium in our series and is often implicated in bacteremia. It is a bacterium that has historically pioneered the epidemic spread of new resistance mechanisms, such as the strains with decreased susceptibility to cephalosporins that were described in Germany in 1983 (30) and the first strain of *K. pneumoniae* showing resistance to imipenem and meropenem described in 2000 in the United States (42).

In our hospital, the problem of *K. pneumoniae* resistance to cefotaxime is still a problem with a slight increase in 11 years from 43% (14) to 52.9% in our series. LART 2014 data reports 45.4% resistance to third generation cephalosporins (10); however, ONERBA in its 2016 report reports 20.7% resistance (28). These results should be stratified according to the providing services and according to the nosocomial or community origin of the infection.

C3G resistance in *K. pneumoniae* is primarily related to the production of CTXM-15 ESBLs (43,44) and these strains are responsible for both nosocomial and community acquired infections (8).

Since 2011, some strains of *K. pneumoniae* have started to show resistance to carbapenems (1.9% resistance to imipenem and ertapenem. This phenomenon rapidly increased to 36.9% resistance in 2015. A study also conducted in our hospital and which concerned the global epidemiology of *K. pneumoniae* strains from 2012 to 2014 found a prevalence of carbapenem resistance equal to 15.8% (45). The Tunisian antibiotic resistance surveillance network reports an overall prevalence of 12.7% of imipenem resistance in *K. pneumoniae*. ONERBA reports the prevalence of 0.1% while the REA-Raisin network talks about 1.6% of carbapenem resistances in enterobacteria in its 2014 report (46).

The use of carbapenems, which are the beta-lactams of last resort in the treatment of severe EBLSE infections, is very often a problem of therapeutic impasse. Indeed, carbapenemase-producing Enterobacteriaceae are often resistant to other classes of antibiotics, particularly fluoroquinolones, aminoglycosides and third-generation cephalosporins, and are therefore real BMRs to be monitored (47).

Resistance of *K. pneumoniae* to carbapenems is primarily due to an enzymatic mechanism consisting of carbapenemase production.

Carbapenemases belong to the Ambler class of beta-lactamases A, B and D. Class A carbapenemases (KPC, IMI, GES) are partially inhibited by clavulanic acid. The KPC enzyme is the most clinically representative of this group. It is inhibited by boronic acid. It is frequently reported in Latin America, the East Coast of the United States and Greece and has also been the cause of several epidemics in Europe. Class B (VIM, IMP, NDM) are metallo-enzymes inhibited by EDTA and dipicolinic acid. They hydrolyze all beta-lactams except aztreonam. Types IMP and VIM are endemic in Greece, Taiwan and Japan. The NDM type, the most recent carbapenemase, has been reported in several countries. Class D carbapenemases type OXA-48 was first described in Turkey and then rapidly spread around the world to become the leading carbapenemase in Mediterranean countries. Their identification is difficult because they are not inhibited by clavulanic acid. They hydrolyze cephalosporins and carbapenems to a small extent but they are often associated with ESBLs; the strains that produce them are therefore often multi-resistant to beta-lactams (48,49). Genotyping of our strains in another study showed that the majority of carbapenem-resistant *K. pneumoniae* produced OXA-48 carbapenemases (45).

The *bla-SHV1* gene is ubiquitous in *K. pneumoniae* and codes for the natural penicillinase of this bacterium. This chromosomal gene has subsequently evolved into a plasmid gene encoding SHV ESBLs (50).

The CA-SFM/EUCAST recommended the use of ertapenem for the detection of carbapenemase-producing strains as it is the most suitable molecule to test for them. It also validated a screening algorithm with 100% sensitivity using ticarcillin-clavulanate, temocillin, and cefepime disks to test for carbapenemase production and thus indicate a confirmatory test (51).

The risk factors for carbapenemase-producing enterobacteria are similar to those that predispose to EBLSE infection, including hospitalization in an intensive care unit, use of a beta-lactam/beta-lactamase inhibitor combination, cephalosporins, fluoroquinolones and urinary catheterization (52).

Enterobacteriaceae and colistin resistance

Colistin resistance in enterobacteria detected in our work was reported in *K. pneumoniae* in 2015. The medical resuscitation service seems the most affected with 3 isolated strains. Nevertheless, the first colistin-resistant strain of *K. pneumoniae was* isolated in our hospital in 2012 from a patient who had been treated with this antibiotic. Others followed to reach 13 strains in five years. The Tunisian LART network detected the first resistances in *K. peumoniae* in 2005 with a prevalence of 0.2%. The trend seems to increase to reach 2.5% in 2014 (10).

Colistin, an antibiotic that has long been neglected because of its renal toxicity, has returned to medical prescriptions as a molecule of last resort in infections with carbapenem-resistant bacteria.

The prevalence of colistin resistance remains low, however, there are variations between countries and there appears to be a correlation with the prevalence of carbapenemase-producing Enterobacteriaceae and thus with the treatment of these infections with colistin (53,54).

The mechanisms of acquired resistance of enterobacteria to colistin are chromosomal or plasmid.

Chromosomal resistance of enterobacteria to colistin results in modifications of LPS to decrease its negative charge necessary for the action of this antibiotic. Other strategies have been described such as the synthesis of a capsule or the synthesis of efflux pumps.

The second mechanism of polymixin resistance is plasmid resistance (53).

In the work performed at our laboratory from 2012 to 2016, sequencing of colistin-resistant *K. pneumoniae did* not find the plasmid resistance genes mcr-1 to mcr-5. All strains had mutations in the mgrB genes (55).

The plasmid resistance mechanism is much more worrying given the possibility of horizontal transfer between different bacterial species. Indeed, the discovery of the *mcr- 1* gene in 2015 in *E. coli* has put the scientific community on alert. However, MICs to colistin in isolates expressing this gene are between 2 and 4 mg/L which confers a low level resistance to polymyxins (53,56). Nevertheless, precautions should be taken, since theoretically it would be sufficient for these strains to acquire a new mechanism of resistance to progress to a high level of resistance.

A. baumannii

It is the number one germ isolated in surgical, medical and POG resuscitation units. It is often responsible for bacteremia, medical device infections and respiratory infections in resuscitation patients.

This non-fermentative Gram-negative bacillus is the very type of pan-resistant or total-resistant bacterium with more than 90% resistance to almost all classes of antibiotics which almost always confronts us with therapeutic impasse. Only colistin and sometimes rifampicin seem to keep an activity, nevertheless the resistance to rifampicin seems to vary according to the years.

A. baumannii is an adaptive model, as it was considered to have low pathogenicity and a multi-susceptible phenotype until the 1970s, when it began to develop several resistance mechanisms and to establish itself as an MRB responsible for several epidemic outbreaks (57).

This bacterium has a natural noninducible cephalosporinase which confers resistance to aminopenicillins, [1st] and [2nd] generation cephalosporins. Like other class C enzymes, it is not inhibited by beta-lactamase inhibitors. *A. baumannii* also possesses a natural chromosomal oxacillinase OXA-51 (class D enzyme), as well as a reduced number of porins which gives it a natural impermeability. This impermeability is also associated with an efflux pump that is active against chloramphenicol and trimethoprim, among others (58). In addition, this MBR has the capacity to acquire several resistance genes, as the *A. baumannii* pan-genome is very large and its size increases exponentially with the sequencing of new genomes; this is referred to as an "open" pan-genome (59).

The carbapenemases described in *A. baumannii* belong to classes A, B (metallo-betalactamases) and D (oxacillinases). Class D carbapenemases or oxacillinases seem to be often involved in the resistance of this bacterium to carbapenems. Although these enzymes confer decreased susceptibility to carbapenems and have limited hydrolysis of extended-spectrum cephalosporins, it is their frequent association with other resistance mechanisms such as efflux and impermeability that is responsible for the high level of resistance to carbapenems (60).

OXA-23 is the most common enzyme and has been reported worldwide; the prevalence of the blaOXA-23 like gene was 93% in bacteremia strains isolated from burn patients in China (61). A Tunisian study of strains from the Institut d'Orthopédie Mohamed Kassab found the blaOXA-23like gene in all isolates (62).

In view of the resistance profile of *A. baumannii* to antibiotics, colistin is now considered as the drug of last resort. Nevertheless, some strains are already showing resistance to this antibiotic.

In our series, colistin resistance was not detected. Nevertheless, the first colistin resistance in *A. baumannii* in our hospital was recently detected in a patient hospitalized in cardiovascular and thoracic surgery (63).

These results probably underestimate the reality of *A. baumannii* resistance to colistin. Indeed, the recommendations of the CA-SFM in 2013 were questioned by the CA-SFM/EUCAST from 2014; it is no longer recommended to use colistin discs or E-test strips to test the susceptibility of a strain, it is the determination of MIC by microdilution in liquid medium that remains the reference method (64).

The resistance of *A. baumannii* to colistin is linked to point mutations in the pmrA and pmrB genes, which reduce the negative charges on the outer membrane of the bacterium necessary for the action of this molecule (60,65). Complete genome sequencing of a strain isolated in our laboratory from a patient treated with colistin, rifampin and amikacin after mitral valve replacement revealed a three-nucleotide duplication in the pmrB gene and a mutation in the rpoB gene (63); this confirms the role of antibiotic pressure in the development of resistance

Pseudomonas aeruginosa

It is the second most common non-fermentative Gram-negative bacillus responsible for nososomal infections in our patients.

Our *P. aeruginosa* strains showed varying rates of resistance to the antibiotics tested. There seems to be an increase in resistance until 2014 and then a clear decrease is observed in 2016, during which year the resistance to imipenem reached 20.6% and the resistances to ceftazidime, piperacillin-tazobactam and ciprofloxacin did not exceed 10%. This is probably due to the hygienic measures implemented in these wards with high risk of nosocomial infections. Nevertheless, the overall trend of resistance to ciprofloxacin, amikacin and beta-lactams, with the exception of ceftazidime, seems to be stable.

ONERBA reports resistance to ceftazidime, piperacillin-tazobactam, imipenem, and ciprofloxacin of 13.2%, 14.1%, 15.3%, and 25.8%, respectively, in its 2016 report (28). The REA Raisin network reports 17.1% resistance to ceftazidime and 19.7% resistance to imipenem in 2014. In the latest report of the Tunisian LART network conducted in 2014, we find 13.2%, 21.1% and 25.1% of resistances to ceftazidime, imipenem and ciprofloxacin respectively (10).

Pseudomonas aeruginosa is naturally resistant to aminopenicillins, 2nd and 3rd generation cephalosporins (cefotaxime and ceftriaxone). This is due to the low permeability of its outer membrane associated with an inducible cephalosporinase ampC and the presence of active efflux pumps.

Resistance to ceftazidime is primarily related to the hyperproduction of the cephalosporinase AmpC, which confers resistance to all beta-lactams except imipenem; however, in some cases, resistance to third-generation cephalosporins may be related to the production of an ESBL belonging to classes A or D.

Resistance to carbapenems in *P. aeruginosa* may be due either to a change in the OprD porin that results in isolated resistance to imipenem or to the production of a carbapenemase. The most frequent carbapenemases are metallo-beta-lactamases (class B). They hydrolyse all beta-lactams except aztreonam. The search for synergy between a disk of imipenem or meropenem combined with EDTA makes it possible to detect carbapenemase-producing strains of the metallo-beta-lactamase type (66). A study of 48 *P. aeruginosa* strains in an intensive care unit in Iran found 75% BMR isolates. Among the carbapenem-resistant strains, the blaIMP and blaVIM genes were found in 31.3% and 14.6% of cases (67). Another study of 21 strains isolated from patients in Libya found the concomitant presence of the blaVIM-2 gene and mutations in the genes encoding oprD porin in all isolates producing a metallo-beta-lactamase (68).

P. aeruginosa is naturally susceptible to ciproloxacin and levofloxacin. Decreased susceptibility to anti-pyocyanine fluoroquinolones may be related to an efflux mechanism (mainly MexAB-OprM and MexXY-OprM) which will also affect other families of antibiotics. Pyocyanins can acquire high level resistance to fluroquinolones which are secondary to mutations in the genes coding for the A subunit of DNA gyrase, or more rarely the B subunit, or for topoisomerase IV. These high-level resistances may also be secondary to the combination of several resistance mechanisms (66). In a Tunisian study of 81 ciprofloxacin-resistant *P. aeruginosa* strains, 77% of isolates had point mutations in both gyrA and parC genes (69).

With its various resistance mechanisms, *P. aeruginosa* seems to have the "qualities" required to join *A. baumannii* among the pan-resistant bacteria. XDR (extensively drug-resistant) clones have already been reported in the literature and are recognised as international high-risk clones (70). Therefore, we need to pay special attention to this germ in order to anticipate the expansion of its antibiotic resistance and its clonal spread.

Enterococcus faecalis

Enterococcus faecalis is the most frequently isolated Gram-positive cocci in our work. It is the most implicated enterococcus in human pathology and is less concerned by the acquisition of antibiotic resistance than *E. faecium*.

Enterococcus faecalis has a PLP5 naturally of low affinity for penicillin G which explains the high MIC of beta-lactams if compared to streptococci. It is naturally resistant to aminoglycosides (low level of resistance), cephalosporins, ertapenem, fluoroquinolones and clindamycin.

E. faecalis keeps a good sensitivity to ampicillin, indeed resistances did not exceed 2.5% during the seven years of our study. The REA Raisin network speaks of 6.7% ampicillin resistance in *E. faecalis* in 2014 (46). The known mechanism of ampicillin resistance is the production of a plasmid penicillinase (71).

High-level resistance to aminoglycosides increased from 15.8% in 2010 to 52.8% in 2015 for gentamicin, which is problematic in case of bacteremia with this germ since the synergistic effect between beta-lactams and aminoglycosides that is sought in this indication is lost. The 2014 LART data report 32.9% of high-level resistance to gentamicin (10). The mechanism of resistance in enterococci is rarely a modification of the ribosomal target, much more often an enzyme synthesis (72).

E. faecalis strains show a high level of resistance to macrolides, with 83.7% and 59.6% of resistance to erythromycin and pristinamycin respectively. The ONERBA reports 70% of strains not sensitive to erythromycin (28).

Resistance to levofloxacin has decreased significantly over these seven years and was eliminated in 2016, which may be due to better prescription of this antibiotic.

Since the year 2013, there is emergence of some glycopeptide resistant strains; this phenomenon has become more widespread in *Enterococcus faecium* species.

The genetic basis for acquired glycopeptide resistance in enterococci is plasmid-based. Five genes have been identified but the VanA gene followed by VanB are the most frequent (73).

Several risk factors for GRI (glycopeptide-resistant enterococci) infection have been identified in the literature, including a stay in an intensive care unit, a history of hospitalization, prolonged hospitalization, the presence of comorbidities, renal failure, neoplasia, a history of surgery, invasive procedures, the presence of foreign material, and previous prescriptions of antibiotics, mainly vancomycin, third-generation cephalosporins, and penicillins. These risk factors are often found in intensive care and urology patients, which should alert us to pay particular attention to these high-risk departments (74).

Staphylococcus aureus

It is the second most common Gram-positive cocci in our study. More than 90% of the strains were resistant to amoxicillin. This result is found in both the LART and ONERBA data (10,28). Indeed, the penicillinase phenotype has become very common in S. aureus both in the hospital and in the community. The percentage of meticillin resistance has gradually increased to reach 20% in 2016. The percentage of overall meticillin resistance was 14.2% in 2015 for France and 22.7% for Tunisia in 2014 (10,28).

In contrast, the REA Raisin network observed a decrease in MRSA (methicillin-resistant Staphylococcus aureus) from 48.7% in 2004 to 19.3% in 2014 (46).

The mechanism of resistance of *S. aureus* to meticillin often involves the acquisition of an exogenous PLP: PLP2a encoded by the mecA gene. The production of PLP2a, which is often inducible, will result in cross-resistance to all beta-lactams (75), and the best therapeutic option is to use glycopeptides.

In 2013 and 2014 we had some vancomycin resistant strains. This coincides with the start of the ERG outbreak in our hospital. Although we have not isolated any glycopeptide resistant *S. aureus* since then, this is indeed a red flag especially as the number of ERGs is expanding. Indeed, the fear of transfer of glycopeptide resistance genes from enterococci to staphylococci has been confirmed in vivo since 2003 (76,77).

Our strains do not express much resistance to aminoglycosides. Gentamicin remains the molecule of choice with 6.7% resistance in 2016. Indeed, the loss of synergy between beta-lactams and gentamicin is due to the production of a single bifunctional enzyme, aminoglycoside acetyltransferase (6')-phosphotransferase (2"). Furthermore, this antibiotic (along with netilmicin) is less frequently affected than other aminoglycosides in MRSA (5-30% resistance) (78).

Intensive care units

The most common bacteriological samples taken in the ICU are blood cultures, ECBU, respiratory samples such as PDP and bronchial suctioning and various medical devices.

The most frequently isolated bacteria are *A. baumannii, P. aeruginosa, K. pneumoniae, E. coli* and *S. aureus*. In our work, *A. baumannii* is the first germ isolated from blood cultures. Bacteremia in intensive care patients are mainly related to two types of infection: ventilator-associated pneumonia (VAP) and urinary tract infections.

These infections are intimately linked to the placement of medical devices; patients are therefore exposed to urinary tract infections, catheter-related bacteremia and VAP.

VAP is the leading cause of nosocomial infection in the ICU with an incidence of between 10 and 40%. This incidence varies according to the intensive care unit and the duration of intubation. The responsible agents are BGN and/or *S. aureus*. In our work, *S. aureus* was the first germ isolated from respiratory samples in the ICU followed by non-fermentative BGN.

The mortality of patients with VAP is high, ranging from 20 to over 65% depending on the study. Certain germs seem to be associated with a better prognosis, such as *P. aeruginosa* (79).

Urinary tract infections are also very frequent in patients hospitalized in the ICU and they occur mainly on urinary catheters. The germs isolated from urine in our work are essentially *E. coli, P. aeruginosa, A. baumannii* and *K. pneumoniae*. However, a positive culture does not systematically mean infection, and this is where clinical-biological collaboration becomes important (80).

For both VAP and UTIs, the diagnosis is based as much on microbiology as on clinical findings. It is important to respect this duality so as not to treat a patient who has a positive respiratory specimen or bacteriuria and who is in fact colonized and not infected. This is essential in terms of health economics but also to avoid the emergence and spread of multi-resistant bacteria due to antibiotic selection pressure.

It is clear that microbiological samples should be taken before initiating or changing antibiotic therapy (79,80).

Hospitalization in the ICU is a risk factor for BMR infection (38,52). The choice of probabilistic antibiotic therapy must therefore be guided by the ecology of the ward, which brings us back to the importance of monitoring the evolution of bacterial resistance to anti-infectives. Antibiotic therapy should then be adapted to the results of the antibiogram in case of positive culture.

The Urology Department

E. coli is the most frequently isolated bacterium from patients hospitalized in the urology department. It is followed by *K. pneumoniae* and *E. faecalis.* The UBE is the most requested type of bacteriological analysis in this department.

Resistance to ³ʳᵈ generation cephalosporins exceeds 20% in *E. coli* and 50% in *K. pneumoniae.*

In 2010, ESBLs were mainly detected in *K. pneumoniae,* but for the last few years, the most problematic BMR in the urology department is cefotaxime-resistant *E. coli* through ESBL production. In a study carried out in our laboratory on ESBL-producing uropathogenic Enterobacteriaceae in the urology department from 2004 to 2008, *K. pneumoniae* was the first species isolated with a prevalence of 56% and the CTX-M15 gene was present in all ESBL-producing strains (9). In a study by the European Section for Infections in Urology that looked at healthcare-associated UTIs in urology patients from 2003 to 2010, *E. coli* was the most frequently isolated germ with a prevalence of 39.7% (81).

Fluoroquinolone resistance in our *E. coli* strains was high (49%), which is probably due to the increased use of fluoroquinolones in this department. M. Cek et al. report that fluoroquinolones were the most prescribed drugs in urology departments (81). Fosfomycin continues to have very good activity with 0.4% of resistance. Its use in prophylaxis in transrectal biopsies of the prostate seems interesting; a meta-analysis has shown that infectious complications in patients who received prophylaxis with fosfomycin-trometamol were significantly rarer than in patients who received prophylaxis with fluoroquinolones (82)

A positive urine culture does not mean infection. Indeed, the majority of urology patients have asymptomatic bacteriuria (9,81). In this case, too, the microbiological result must be interpreted according to the clinical context, since colonization of the urine should not be treated except in certain cases, such as in pregnant women or before urinary tract surgery (83).

Urological inpatients are frequently exposed to risk factors for EBLSE, which include prior antibiotic therapy, urological history, renal failure, anemia, unbalanced diabetes, length of hospitalization, bladder catheterization, and drainage time greater than three days (9).

In addition to EBLSE, glycopeptide-resistant enterococci and carbapenemase-producing *K. pneumoniae are* emerging. Although their prevalence is still low, there is a real risk of expansion and dissemination of these emerging BMR among patients hospitalized in the urology department and to other clinical departments. Measures are therefore necessary to face and control the epidemic.

Prevention of the spread of BMR :

The prevention of the spread of BMR in high-risk departments is based on close collaboration between the microbiology laboratory, the operational hygiene team, the clinical departments, the pharmacy and the Committee for the Control of Nosocomial Infections (CLIN).

The role of the microbiology laboratory is essential because it is the laboratory that identifies BMR, performs antibiograms, searches for the resistance genes responsible for the observed phenotype, and looks for clonality between strains from different departments in order to understand how a BMR spreads. It also plays a role in the epidemiological surveillance of the evolution of bacterial resistance to antibiotics. It keeps the clinical departments informed of their bacterial ecology in order to guide the initiation of probabilistic treatments and provides them with statistics relating to each department.

When isolating an MRB, it is the speed of response that will make the difference (84,85). The microbiology laboratory quickly informs the relevant clinical department and the operational hygiene team. If more than two cases of infection with the same species and resistance pattern are found, an outbreak is suspected and urgent action should be taken (85).

Hygienists have a crucial role in prevention and intervention. They ensure that standard hygiene precautions are applied, as they are unfortunately often neglected by healthcare workers and patients. The French Society of Hospital Hygiene has recently published an update on standard precautions, in which it emphasizes the importance of hand washing in preventing cross-transmission of germs, and that these measures should be applied to everyone (patient and professional), for all care and for all places (86). In the event of an epidemic or isolation of a BMR, hygienists have an intervention role by visiting the clinical department concerned to ensure that additional precautions are implemented, such as contact precautions and isolation if possible (84).

At the Sahloul University Hospital, the prevention and safety of care service, formerly named hospital hygiene service, has as its main mission (in collaboration with the CLIN) the prevention of infections associated with care (IAS). In addition to the regular activities of monitoring, control and control of HCAI, the entire team of this service has been engaged (with the hospital management) since 2015 in a policy of implementation of the multimodal strategy of hand hygiene promotion recommended by the WHO. The activities carried out within the framework of this strategy have mainly concerned:

- *The realization of training sessions for hospital staff to remind them of the role of hand hygiene in the prevention of HCAI, the indications and techniques of hand washing and hydro-alcoholic friction.*

- *Reporting the results of the hand hygiene compliance audit carried out as part of this strategy*

- *Updating and disseminating communication and awareness materials related to good hand hygiene practices.*

This action may partly explain the slight improvement in BMR numbers seen between the years 2014 and 2016 for some bacteria.

The spread of highly resistant bacteria or HRB (carbapenemase-producing enterobacteria and glycopeptide-resistant enterococci) is sporadic or epidemic. Enterococci and enterobacteria are part of the intestinal microbiota, so these HRB pose the problem of digestive carriage, which may be prolonged, given that we do not yet have effective means of decontamination (84).

A. baumannii and *P. aeruginosa* are saprophytic bacteria that infect patients with special conditions, such as intensive care patients. It is becoming increasingly clear that transmission occurs through surfaces contaminated with these bacteria. For this reason, proper cleaning of surfaces must be part of the measures to prevent the spread of BMR (87).

The second axis of the fight against antibiotic resistance is represented by the rules of good antibiotic use or "Antibiotic Stewardship". Indeed, the emergence of new resistance phenotypes generally follows the marketing of a new antibiotic. It is therefore in order to spare the molecules of last resort that we must improve the consumption of antibiotics. In the microbiology laboratory of the Sahloul Hospital, we systematically provide a copy to the pharmacy of the antibiograms performed for each positive sample from hospitalized patients. This makes it possible to some extent to adjust prescriptions based on antibiotic susceptibility tests.

An audit, conducted by the hygiene department and the microbiology laboratory among physicians in our hospital, assessed perceptions, knowledge and attitudes regarding bacterial resistance and antibiotic prescribing. It showed that knowledge about the prevalence of bacterial resistance and antibiotic misuse was poor (88).

The reactivation of existing structures such as the CLIN and the creation of an antibiotics committee therefore seem justified in view of the problems of growth of bacterial resistance that we observe. This committee should be made up of at least one microbiologist, one hygienist, one pharmacist and one infectiologist. A referent in antibiotic therapy should be present in each clinical department to collaborate with this team. Antibiotic stewardship interventions appear to be successful; indeed, a German team recently published the results of an interventional study and demonstrated that there was a clear reduction in resistance of enterobacteria to C3Gs and a reduction in antibiotic consumption (89).

At the Sahloul University Hospital, currently, within the framework of the project to support the competitiveness of services (PACS) with a view to setting up a quality and risk management system, a process to reactivate the various committees such as the CLIN, the therapeutic committee and others has been launched by the hospital's medical committee. The results of the work of these committees will certainly have a positive impact on the evolution of BMR rates. The latter will be the subject of possible impact studies or evaluation of actions and measures implemented in this perspective.

Another approach to controlling the transmission of BMRs in patients with risk factors is vaccination. Influenza vaccination has been associated with fewer infections with BMRs since bacterial superinfection and MVAP in patients with malignant influenza are important complications in this case. There are also vaccines in development to prevent *Clostridium difficile* and *S. aureus* infections. Perhaps in a few years vaccines will also be developed that prevent *GRE* or *A. baumannii* infections, which would allow us to identify patients with risk factors for BMR infection and prevent these infections altogether through vaccination (90).

Conclusion

Conclusion:

Bacterial resistance to antibiotics, a real and constantly evolving public health problem, is a real pandemic and concerns both the hospital and the community environment.

The WHO has made this a stated priority; In the most recent of its reports, February 2017, it published a list of resistant bacteria for which there is an urgent need to develop a new therapeutic strategy, if necessary new antibiotic molecules.

Our country is also concerned by the increase of antibiotic resistance of bacteria. The Tunisian network LART gathers several microbiology laboratories in order to monitor the evolution of these resistances.

The microbiology laboratory plays an essential role in the detection of resistance mechanisms and in the prevention of the spread of BMR in collaboration with the clinical services and the hygiene service. Our hospital, which has a surgical vocation, is particularly concerned by the problem of bacterial resistance to antibiotics, given the frequency of infections associated with care and particularly nosocomial infections. It is within this framework that we carried out this work which aims to describe the bacterial ecology of four services at risk of nosocomial infections in our hospital and to determine the level of resistance of the principal isolated species.

Therefore, we conducted a retrospective descriptive study of all non-redundant strains isolated from patients hospitalized in the urology, surgical resuscitation, medical resuscitation and POG departments. The study period was from January 1, 2010 to December 31, 2016. For each strain, we noted the antibiotic resistance profile, the requesting department, the type of specimen and the year of isolation.

The Chi-square test was used to compare trends in the annual percentages of resistance for the most representative antibiotic/bacterial species pairs. It was also used to look for a significant increase in fluoroquinolone and aminoglycoside resistance in cefotaxime-resistant strains. A total of 6108 non-redundant bacterial strains were isolated over a seven-year period. The most frequent bacteria were *E. coli* (21.8%), *K. pneumoniae* (16.2%), *A. baumannii* (12.5%), *P. aeruginosa* (10.2%), *E. faecalis* (7.8%) and *S. aureus* (6%).

The most frequent source was the urology department with 43.4% of isolates. The most frequent samples were ECBU (45.8%), blood cultures (22.4%), medical devices (8.9%) and PDP (8.9%).

We noticed significant differences in the bacterial resistance of the main species isolated in different years.

In *E. coli,* the trend was for increasing resistance to amoxicillin, amoxicillin-clavulanate, cefotaxime, gentamicin, fluoroquinolones and cotrimoxazole. Resistance to cefotaxime reached 38.7% of strains in 2016. During the study period, two strains resistant to ertapenem were isolated and no resistance to colistin was noted.

In *K. pneumoniae,* cefotaxime resistance appeared to be stable but resistance to imipenem and gentamicin tended to increase. The first six colistin-resistant strains of *K. pneumoniae were* isolated in 2015.

There was also a significant increase in fluoroquinolone and aminoglycoside resistance in cefotaxime-resistant strains of *K. pneumoniae* and *E. coli*.

A. baumannii was the typical example of BMR with resistances exceeding 90% for most antibiotics. Nevertheless, the two molecules that seemed to retain activity were colistin and rifampicin.

Colistin resistance was probably underestimated as the disc and E-test MIC methods used in our work are no longer recommended by the CA-SFM/EUCAST. Indeed, the MIC measurement by liquid dilution has become the reference method.

P. aeruginosa seems to keep a certain stability regarding antibiotic resistance and the trend seems to be decreasing for ceftazidime resistance during the last three years of the study. This is related to the hygienic measures that have been applied in the departments concerned.

There appears to be an increase in meticillin resistance in *S. aureus from* 11.1% in 2010 to 20% in 2016.

E. faecalis still retains an excellent sensitivity to ampicillin with 1 to 3 resistant strains isolated per year. Nevertheless, there is a trend towards increasing resistance to kanamycin and rifampin. Glycopeptide resistance has also emerged in our hospital with the isolation of two glycopeptide resistant strains of *E. faecalis during* the study period.

The most problematic BMRs in our hospital are non-fermenting Gram-negative bacilli with carbapenem-resistant *A. baumannii* in the intensive care units and ESBL enterobacteria in urology. Cefotaxime-resistant *K. pneumoniae* have been overtaken by cefotaxime-resistant *E. coli*. Since the year 2011, we have observed the emergence and then the increase in the prevalence of ertapenem-resistant *K. pneumoniae*. Since the year 2012, the number of isolated MRSA has also increased. In 2013, the first glycopeptide-resistant *E. faecalis* strain was isolated in the urology department.

E. coli was the first bacterium isolated in the urology department and was mainly from urine. In this department, *E. coli was* resistant to cefotaxime, ertapenem and ciprofloxacin in 21.4%, 0.2% and 49% of cases respectively. *K. pneumoniae* was the second most common enterobacterium isolated and showed 51.4% resistance to cefotaxime, 7.4% resistance to ertapenem and 63.3% resistance to ciprofloxacin. One colistin-resistant strain was reported.

P. aeruginosa strains isolated from the urology department were resistant to ceftazidime, imipenem and ciprofloxacin in 40.6%, 10.3% and 61.2% of cases respectively. No resistance to colistin was noted.

In all three ICUs, blood cultures were the most frequently performed bacteriological test, followed by respiratory, urine and medical device specimens. *A. baumannii was the* most frequent BMR. It was isolated mainly from blood cultures, medical devices and respiratory specimens. In the ICU setting, VAP, catheter infections and urinary tract infections are the most frequent nosocomial infections. *S. aureus is the* germ most incriminated in respiratory infections in the ICU in our work.

We conclude that bacterial resistance to antibiotics is a dynamic and very rapidly evolving phenomenon in our hospital.

The most frequent BMRs in the departments studied are ESBL- and carbapenemase-producing Enterobacteriaceae, and they are mainly isolated from the urology department. In the ICU, multidrug-resistant *A. baumannii* infections are the main problem. The emergence of strains resistant to colistin, which is the antibiotic of last resort, has serious repercussions including therapeutic impasse and the risk of intra- and inter-departmental diffusion.

The emergence of glycopeptide resistance in enterococci must be controlled in order to contain the epidemic and avoid dissemination to the community and transfer of resistance genes to staphylococci.

Monitoring of bacterial resistance to antibiotics by the microbiology laboratory would have more impact if it were done within the CLIN or an antibiotic committee that, based on the report from the microbiology laboratory, could identify priorities for action and key services to be targeted. This committee would consist of a microbiologist, pharmacist, hygienist, infectious disease specialist, and any other health care personnel with an interest in the proper use of antibiotics. This committee should work with clinical departments to improve the prescribing of anti-infective drugs and thus limit the selection of resistant germs through the pressure of these molecules.

It is essential to reactivate existing structures such as the CLIN given the frequency and severity of nosocomial infections in our hospital and the rapid spread of BMR.

It is important that local surveillance of antibiotic resistance be done within the framework of national surveillance in order to have nationwide data. Learned societies should encourage hospital and community laboratories to join and expand existing networks such as LART.

A collective effort must be made to boost this network and have updated annual data, indeed we have no national data since 2014. This is necessary in view of the rapid evolution of bacterial resistance profiles to antibiotics and the rapid appearance and diffusion of new resistance mechanisms.

It is also important to stratify these data according to clinical settings. Community and nosocomial settings are not the same ecology, so it is preferable to have databases specific to each setting to avoid biased figures.

Antibiotic resistance and antimicrobial resistance concern not only healthcare professionals but also the general public, whom we must raise awareness of the dangers of self-medication, particularly in the field of antibiotic therapy.

Collective national and international collaboration to combat the spread of BMRs and to establish rules for the proper use of antibiotics remains the only bulwark against the therapeutic impasse and the risk of returning to the pre-antibiotic era.

Bibliography

Bibliography

1. Moellering RC. Past, present, and future of antimicrobial agents. Am J Med. 1995 Dec 29;99(6A):11S-18S.

2. Fleming A. On the Antibacterial Action of Cultures of a Penicillium, with Special Reference to their Use in the Isolation of B. influenzæ. Br J Exp Pathol. June 1929;10(3):226-36.

3. Gould K. Antibiotics: from prehistory to the present day. J Antimicrob Chemother. march 2016;71(3):572-5.

4. Armand-Lefèvre L. Resistance in the city, myth or reality? The threat of ESBL-producing enterobacteria. J Anti-Infect. 1 March 2017;19(1):1-6.

5. WHO-GLOBAL P RIORITY LIST OF ANTIBIOTIC - RESISTANT BACTERIA TO GUIDE RESEARCH, D ISCOVERY, AND DEVELO PMENT OF NEW ANTIBIOTICS_25 Feb 2017.pdf [Internet]. [cited 13 Jan 2018]. Available from: http://www.who.int/medicines/publications/WHO-PPL-Short_Summary_25Feb-ET_NM_WHO.pdf?ua=1

6. U.S. Antibiotic Awareness Week | U.S. Antibiotic Awareness Week | CDC [Internet]. 2017 [cited 23 Jan 2018]. Available from: https://www.cdc.gov/antibiotic-use/week/index.html

7. Aziza Messaoudi. Study of the molecular basis of beta-lactam resistance in Klebsiella pneumoniae isolated at Sahloul-Sousse hospital. Faculty of Pharmacy of Monastir; 2017.

8. Mansour W, Grami R, Ben Haj Khalifa A, Dahmen S, Châtre P, Haenni M, et al. Dissemination of multidrug-resistant blaCTX-M-15/IncFIIk plasmids in Klebsiella pneumoniae isolates from hospital- and community-acquired human infections in Tunisia. Diagn Microbiol Infect Dis. Nov 2015;83(3):298-304.

9. Habiba Naija. Analytical study of urinary tract infections with extended-spectrum betalactamase-forming bacteria in the urology department and control strategy. Faculty of Medicine of Sousse. 2010.

10. Antibiotic resistance in Tunisia (LART). Data 2012-2014.

11. Picot S, Rakotomalala RS, Farny K, Simac C, Michault A. [Evolution of resistance to antibiotics from 1997 to 2005 in the Reunion Island]. Med Mal Infect. Nov 2010;40(11):617-24.

12. CASFM / EUCAST: French Society of Microbiology Ed; 2017.

13. Magiorakos A-P, Srinivasan A, Carey RB, Carmeli Y, Falagas ME, Giske CG, et al. Multidrug-resistant, extensively drug-resistant and pandrug-resistant bacteria: an

international expert proposal for interim standard definitions for acquired resistance. Clin Microbiol Infect. 2012 Mar 1;18(3):268-81.

14. Salah Jday. Bacterial ecology of BMR in Sahloul hospital of Sousse during the years (2001 to 2005). Faculty of Medicine of Sousse. 2007.docx.

15. CASFM : French Society of Microbiology Ed ; 2010.

16. CASFM: French Society of Microbiology Ed; 2011.

17. CASFM: French Society of Microbiology Ed; 2012.

18. CASFM: French Society of Microbiology Ed; 2013.

19. CASFM / EUCAST: French Society of Microbiology Ed; 2014.

20. CASFM / EUCAST: French Society of Microbiology Ed; 2015.

21. CASFM / EUCAST: French Society of Microbiology Ed; 2016.

22. Bruno Grandbastien, Jérôme Robert. Methodology for monitoring resistance of microorganisms to anti-infectives. In: Rémic Référentiel en Microbiologie Médicale. 5th edition 2015. Société Française de Microbiologie; p. 347-58.

23. BMR-Raisin Network - Results 2013. Surveillance of multidrug-resistant bacteria in French healthcare institutions . pdf.

24. Lachassinne E, Letamendia-Richard E, Gaudelus J. Epidemiology of nosocomial infections in neonatology. Arch Pediatrics. March 1, 2004;11(3):229-33.

25. Multidrug-resistant bacteria: enterobacteriaceae EBLSE on the rise, MRSA staphylococci on the decline [Internet]. Medscape. [cited 2018 Jan 24]. Available from: http://francais.medscape.com/viewarticle/3406253

26. Maoulainine F-M-R, Elidrissi N-S, Chkil G, Abba F, Soraa N, Chabaa L, et al. Epidemiology of bacterial nosocomial infection in a Moroccan neonatal intensive care unit. Arch Pediatrics. Sep 1, 2014;21(9):938-43.

27. Kooli I, Kadri Y, Ben Abdallah H, Mhalla S, Haddad O, Noomen S, et al. Epidemiology of multidrug-resistant bacteria in a Tunisian neonatal unit. J Pediatrics Childcare. Oct 1, 2014;27(5):236-42.

28. ONERBA France. National Observatory of the Epidemiology of Bacterial Resistance to Antibiotics. Rapport d'activi.

29. R. Bonnet. Beta-lactams and enterobacteria. In: P. Courvalin. Antibiogramme. Paris. Editions ESKA/2006, PP141-162.

30. Philippon A. Extended or broad spectrum beta-lactamases (ESBLs). Immuno-Anal

Biol Spec. 1 Oct 2013;28(5):287-96.

31. Bradford PA. Extended-Spectrum p-Lactamases in the 21st Century: Characterization, Epidemiology, and Detection of This Important Resistance Threat. Clin Microbiol Rev. Oct 2001;14(4):933-51.

32. Ayari K, Bourouis A, Chihi H, Mahrouki S, Naas T, Belhadj O. Dissemination and genetic support of broad-spectrum beta-lactam-resistant Escherichia coli strain isolated from two Tunisian hospitals during 2004-2012. Afr Health Sci. June 2017;17(2):346-55.

33. Tayh G, Ben Sallem R, Ben Yahia H, Gharsa H, Klibi N, Boudabous A, et al. First report of extended-spectrum p-lactamases among clinical isolates of Escherichia coli in Gaza Strip, Palestine. J Glob Antimicrob Resist. sept 2016;6:17-21.

34. Dahmen S, Bettaieb D, Mansour W, Boujaafar N, Bouallègue O, Arlet G. Characterization and molecular epidemiology of extended-spectrum beta-lactamases in clinical isolates of Enterobacteriaceae in a Tunisian University Hospital. Microb Drug Resist Larchmt N. June 2010;16(2):163-70.

35. Mnif B, Harhour H, Jdidi J, Mahjoubi F, Genel N, Arlet G, et al. Molecular epidemiology of extended-spectrum beta-lactamase-producing Escherichia coli in Tunisia and characterization of their virulence factors and plasmid addiction systems. BMC Microbiol. 25 June 2013;13:147.

36. Sbiti M, Lahmadi khalid, louzi L. Epidemiological profile of extended-spectrum beta-lactamase-producing uropathogenic enterobacteria. Pan Afr Med J [Internet]. 13 Sep 2017 [cited 3 Jan 2018]; 28. Available from: https://www.ncbi.nlm.nih.gov/pmc/articles/PMC5681015/

37. Sana F, Mabrouka S, Claudine Q, Faouzi SA, Ilhem BBB, Véronique D. Prevalence and characterization of uropathogenic Escherichia coli harboring plasmid-mediated quinolone resistance in a Tunisian university hospital. Diagn Microbiol Infect Dis. 1 June 2014;79(2):247-51.

38. Rodriguez-Bano J, Picon E, Gijon P, Hernandez JR, Ruiz M, Pena C, et al. Community-onset Bacteremia Due to Extended-Spectrum p-Lactamase-Producing Escherichia coli: Risk Factors and Prognosis. Clin Infect Dis. 2010 Jan 1;50(1):40-8.

39. Grami R, Dahmen S, Mansour W, Mehri W, Haenni M, Aouni M, et al. blaCTX-M-15-Carrying F2:A-:B- Plasmid in Escherichia coli from Cattle Milk in Tunisia. Microb Drug Resist. 15 Jan 2014;20(4):344-9.

40. Grami R, Mansour W, Dahmen S, Mehri W, Haenni M, Aouni M, et al. The blaCTX-M-1 IncI1/ST3 plasmid is dominant in chickens and pets in Tunisia. J Antimicrob Chemother. 1 Dec 2013;68(12):2950-2.

41. Grover SS, Doda A, Gupta N, Gandhoke I, Batra J, Hans C, et al. New Delhi metallo-p-

lactamase - type carbapenemases producing Escherichia coli isolates from hospitalized patients: A pilot study. Indian J Med Res. Jul 2017;146(1):105-10.

42. Yigit H, Queenan AM, Anderson GJ, Domenech-Sanchez A, Biddle JW, Steward CD, et al. Novel carbapenem-hydrolyzing beta-lactamase, KPC-1, from a carbapenem-resistant strain of Klebsiella pneumoniae. Antimicrob Agents Chemother. Apr 2001;45(4):1151-61.

43. Alibi S, Ferjani A, Boukadida J. Molecular characterization of extended spectrum beta-lactamases produced by Klebsiella pneumoniae clinical strains from a Tunisian Hospital. Med Mal Infect. Apr 2015;45(4):139-43.

44. Doi Y, Iovleva A, Bonomo RA. The ecology of extended-spectrum p-lactamases (ESBLs) in the developed world. J Travel Med. 1 Apr 2017;24(suppl_1):S44-51.

45. Aziza Messaoudi. Study of the molecular basis of beta-lactam resistance in Klebsiella pneumoniae isolated at .

46. Surveillance of nososomal infections in adult intensive care units. Réseau REA-Raisin, France-Résultats 2014.

47. European Centre for Disease Prevention and Control. Summary of the last data on antibiotic resistance in the European Union.

48. Nordmann P, Naas T, Poirel L. Global spread of Carbapenemase-producing Enterobacteriaceae. Emerg Infect Dis. Oct 2011;17(10):1791-8.

49. Nordmann P, Carrer A. Carbapenemases of enterobacteria. /data/revues/0929693X/v17sS4/S0929693X10709180/ [Internet]. Sep 7, 2010 [cited 2018 Jan 4]; Available from: http://www.em-consulte.com/en/article/264877

50. Stürenburg E, Mack D. Extended-spectrum beta-lactamases: implications for the clinical microbiology laboratory, therapy, and infection control. J Infect. Nov 2003;47(4):273-95.

51. French Society of Microbiology. Phenotypic algorithm for the screening of ca.-producing Enterobacteriaceae strains.

52. Wang Z, Qin R-R, Huang L, Sun L-Y. Risk Factors for Carbapenem-resistant Klebsiella pneumoniae Infection and Mortality of Klebsiella pneumoniae Infection. Chin Med J (Engl). 5 Jan 2018;131(1):56-62.

53. Dortet L, Bonnin R, Jousset A, Gauthier L, Naas T. Emergence of colistin resistance in Enterobacteriaceae: a breach in the last bulwark against pan-resistance! J Anti-Infect. 1 Dec 2016;18(4):139-59.

54. Wertheim H, Van Nguyen K, Hara GL, Gelband H, Laxminarayan R, Mouton J, et al.

Global survey of polymyxin use: A call for international guidelines. J Glob Antimicrob Resist. 1 Sep 2013;1(3):131-4.

55. Jaidane N, Bonnin RA, Mansour W, Girlich D, Creton E, Colleton G, et al. Genomic insights into Colistin-resistant Klebsiella pneumoniae from a Tunisian teaching hospital. Antimicrob Agents Chemother. 11 Dec 2017;

56. Liu Y-Y, Wang Y, Walsh TR, Yi L-X, Zhang R, Spencer J, et al. Emergence of plasmid-mediated colistin resistance mechanism MCR-1 in animals and human beings in China: a microbiological and molecular biological study. Lancet Infect Dis. Feb 2016;16(2):161-8.

57. Marie-Laure JOLY-GUILLOU. Acinetobacter. In: P. Courvalin. Antibiogramme. Paris. Editions ESKA/2006, PP395-406.

58. Decré D. Acinetobacter baumannii and antibiotic resistance: A model of adaptation. Rev Francoph Lab. Apr 1, 2012;2012(441J:43-52.

59. Antunes LCS, Visca P, Towner KJ. Acinetobacter baumannii: evolution of a global pathogen. Pathog Dis. Aug 2014;71(3J:292-301.

60. Poirel L, Bonnin RA, Nordmann P. Genetic basis of antibiotic resistance in pathogenic Acinetobacter species. IUBMB Life. Dec 2011;63(12J:1061-7.

61. Huang G, Yin S, Xiang L, Gong Y, Sun K, Luo X, et al. Epidemiological characterization of Acinetobacter baumannii bloodstream isolates from a Chinese Burn Institute: A three-year study. Burns J Int Soc Burn Inj. Nov 2016;42(7J:1542-7.

62. Mathlouthi N, Ben Lamine Y, Somai R, Bouhalila-Besbes S, Bakour S, Rolain J-M, et al. Incidence of OXA-23 and OXA-58 Carbapenemases Coexpressed in Clinical Isolates of Acinetobacter baumannii in Tunisia. Microb Drug Resist Larchmt N. 10 Jul 2017;

63. Jaidane N, Naas T, Mansour W, Radhia BB, Jerbi S, Boujaafar N, et al. Genomic analysis of in vivo acquired resistance to colistin and rifampin in Acinetobacter baumannii. Int J Antimicrob Agents [Internet]. 7 Nov 2017 [cited 5 Jan 2018]; 0(0J. Available from: http://www.ijaaonline.com/article/S0924-8579f17J30389-8/fulltext

64. French Society of Microbiology. Acinetobacter spp. In: CASFM/EUCAST: Société Française de Microbiologie Ed; 2014 : p.

65. Adams MD, Nickel GC, Bajaksouzian S, Lavender H, Murthy AR, Jacobs MR, et al. Resistance to Colistin in Acinetobacter baumannii Associated with Mutations in the PmrAB Two-Component System. Antimicrob Agents Chemother. 2009 Sep;53(9J:3628-34.

66. Mérens A, Janvier F, Vu-Thien H, Cavallo J-D, Jeannot K. Antibiotic resistance phenotypes of Pseudomonas aeruginosa, Stenotrophomonas maltophilia,

Burkholderia cepacia. Rev Francoph Lab. 1 Sep 2012;2012(445J:59-74.

67. Khorvash F, Yazdani M, Shabani S, Soudi A. Pseudomonas aeruginosa-producing Metallo-p-lactamases (VIM, IMP, SME, and AIMJ in the Clinical Isolates of Intensive Care Units, a University Hospital in Isfahan, Iran. Adv Biomed Res. 2017;6:147.

68. Mathlouthi N, Areig Z, Al Bayssari C, Bakour S, Ali El Salabi A, Ben Gwierif S, et al. Emergence of Carbapenem-Resistant Pseudomonas aeruginosa and Acinetobacter baumannii Clinical Isolates Collected from Some Libyan Hospitals. Microb Drug Resist. 14 Jan 2015;21(3J:335-41.

69. Ben Nejma M, Sioud O, Mastouri M. Quinolone-resistant clinical strains of Pseudomonas aeruginosa isolated from University Hospital in Tunisia. 3 Biotech. jan 2018;8(1J:1.

70. Cabot G, Ocampo-Sosa AA, Dominguez MA, Gago JF, Juan C, Tubau F, et al. Genetic Markers of Widespread Extensively Drug-Resistant Pseudomonas aeruginosa High-Risk Clones. Antimicrob Agents Chemother. dec 2012;56(12):6349-57.

71. J. L. MAINARDI. Beta-lactams and enterococci. In: P. Courvalin. Antibiogramme. Paris. Editions ESKA/2006, p.133-139.

72. R. Bismuth. Aminosides and Gram-positive bacteria. In: P. Courvalin. Antibiogramme. Paris. Editions ESKA/2006, p205-225.

73. Ahmed MO, Baptiste KE. Vancomycin-Resistant Enterococci: A Review of Antimicrobial Resistance Mechanisms and Perspectives of Human and Animal Health. Microb Drug Resist Larchmt N. 23 Oct 2017;

74. Monteserin N, Larson E. Temporal trends and risk factors for healthcare-associated vancomycin-resistant enterococci in adults. J Hosp Infect. nov 2016;94(3):236-41.

75. H. B. Drugeon. Beta-lactams and Staphylococci. In: P. Courvalin. Antibiogramme. Paris. Editions ESKA/2006, p117-124.

76. Chang S, Sievert DM, Hageman JC, Boulton ML, Tenover FC, Downes FP, et al. Infection with Vancomycin-Resistant Staphylococcus aureus Containing the vanA Resistance Gene. N Engl J Med. 3 Apr 2003;348(14):1342-7.

77. Périchon B, Courvalin P. VanA-Type Vancomycin-Resistant Staphylococcus aureus. Antimicrob Agents Chemother. Nov 2009;53(11):4580-7.

78. Leclercq R. Resistance of staphylococci to antibiotics. Ann Fr Anesth Réanimation. 1 May 2002;21(5):375-83.

79. J.- L. TROUILLET et al. Pneumonia acquired under mechanical ventilation. In: Infectiology in intensive care. Springer-Verlag France. Paris; 2013. p. 407-22.

80. Auboyer C. Urinary tract infections in the ICU: diagnosis and treatment /data/revues/0399077x/v0033i09/03001513/ [Internet]. [cited 14 Jan 2018]; Available from: http://www.em-consulte.com/en/article/17589

81. Cek M, Tandogdu Z, Wagenlehner F, Tenke P, Naber K, Bjerklund-Johansen TE. Healthcare-associated urinary tract infections in hospitalized urological patients--a global perspective: results from the GPIU studies 2003-2010. World J Urol. Dec 2014;32(6):1587-94.

82. Roberts MJ, Scott S, Harris PN, Naber K, Wagenlehner FME, Doi SAR. Comparison of fosfomycin against fluoroquinolones for transrectal prostate biopsy prophylaxis: an individual patient-data meta-analysis. World J Urol. 29 Dec 2017;

83. Asymptomatic bacteriuria. Definitions, Conduct To Be Taken | Urofrance [Internet]. [cited 16 Jan 2018]. Available from: http://www.urofrance.org/nc/science-et-research/base-bibliography/article/html/bacteriuria-asymptomatic-definitions-conduit-a-tenir.html

84. Lepelletier D, Batard E, Berthelot P, Zahar J-R, Lucet J-C, Fournier S, et al [Carbapenemase-producing enterobacteriae: epidemiology, strategies to control their spread and issues]. Rev Med Interne. Jul 2015;36(7):474-9.

85. Steinmann J, Kaase M, Gatermann S, Popp W, Steinmann E, Damman M, et al. Outbreak due to a Klebsiella pneumoniae strain harbouring KPC-2 and VIM-1 in a German university hospital, July 2010 to January 2011. Euro Surveill Bull Eur Sur Mal Transm Eur Commun Dis Bull. 18 August 2011;16(33).

86. French Society of Hospital Hygiene. Update of Standard Precautions [Internet]. SF2H. 2017 [cited 17 Jan 2018]. Available from: https://sf2h.net/publications/actualisation-precautions-standard-2017

87. Gandra S, Ellison RT. Modern trends in infection control practices in intensive care units. J Intensive Care Med. Dec 2014;29(6):311-26.

88. M. Ben Rejeb, M. Ben Fredj, B. Kacem, S. Khefacha-Aissa, O. Bouallègue, L. Dhidah, et al. Bacterial resistance and antibiotic prescription: Perceptions, attitudes and knowledge of Tunisian hospital doctors. Rev Tunis D'Infectiologie. 22 Sep 2014;Jan-Apr 2015, Vol.9(N°1/2):17-24.

89. Bonsignore M, Balamitsa E, Nobis C, Tafelski S, Geffers C, Nachtigall I. [Antibiotic stewardship in a basic care hospital: A retrospective observational study]. Anaesthesist. 2 Jan 2018;

90. Jansen KU, Knirsch C, Anderson AS. The role of vaccines in preventing bacterial antimicrobial resistance. Nat Med. 9 Jan 2018;24(1):10-9.

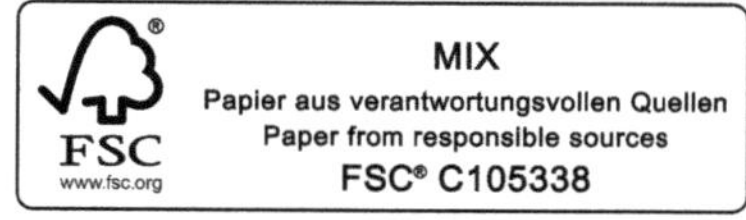